Novel Challenges and Therapeutic Options for Digestive and Liver Diseases

Novel Challenges and Therapeutic Options for Digestive and Liver Diseases

Guest Editors

Daniel Paramythiotis
Eleni Karlafti

MDPI

Basel • Beijing • Wuhan • Barcelona • Belgrade • Novi Sad • Cluj • Manchester

Guest Editors

Daniel Paramythiotis
First Propaedeutic Surgical Department
Aristotle University of Thessaloniki
Thessaloniki
Greece

Eleni Karlafti
Emergency Department
Aristotle University of Thessaloniki
Thessaloniki
Greece

Editorial Office
MDPI AG
Grosspeteranlage 5
4052 Basel, Switzerland

This is a reprint of the Special Issue, published open access by the journal *Journal of Personalized Medicine* (ISSN 2075-4426), freely accessible at: https://www.mdpi.com/journal/jpm/special_issues/0BCZE8LR5V.

For citation purposes, cite each article independently as indicated on the article page online and as indicated below:

Lastname, A.A.; Lastname, B.B. Article Title. *Journal Name* **Year**, *Volume Number*, Page Range.

ISBN 978-3-7258-5505-6 (Hbk)
ISBN 978-3-7258-5506-3 (PDF)
https://doi.org/10.3390/books978-3-7258-5506-3

Contents

About the Editors

Daniel Paramythiotis

Daniel Paramythiotis graduated from the Medical School of Aristotle University of Thessaloniki in 1994 and received his PhD degree in 2002 (grade Excellent). He was recognized as a Specialist General Surgeon in 2002, and he holds a postgraduate diploma specializing in liver–biliary–pancreatic surgery from the School of Medicine of the Democritus University of Thrace. Additionally, he is an instructor on the postgraduate trauma management program (A.T.L.S.) of Northern Greece. He trained at the University Surgery Clinics of Heidelberg and Munich, as well as at St Mark's Hospital in London, participating in major surgeries of the pancreas, liver, esophagus, and colon. Daniel is a Full Professor of Surgery in the First Propaedeutic Department of Surgery, AHEPA University General Hospital, Aristotle University of Thessaloniki, Greece. Also, he is a member of the Disciplinary Board of the Medical Society of Thessaloniki, and he served as member of the Board of Directors of the AHEPA University Hospital of Thessaloniki, member of the Scientific Council of the AHEPA University Hospital of Thessaloniki, member of the General Assembly of School of Medicine of Aristotle University of Thessaloniki, and member of the Committee of the Office of Education of the School of Medicine of Aristotle University of Thessaloniki. His long-term service in a university clinic and his unique abilities have resulted in his remarkable writing and research work, with numerous publications in Greek and international medical journals. Daniel has been recognized with numerous awards, and he is frequently a speaker at conferences and on post-educational courses.

Eleni Karlafti

Eleni Karlafti graduated from the Medical School of Aristotle University of Thessaloniki in 2007 and received her PhD degree in Hypertension and Obesity in 2016 (grade Excellent). In 2021, she received her MSc degree in "New methods and technologies in treatment of Diabetes Mellitus". Eleni was recognized as an Internal Medicine Specialist in 2017, awarded as a Hypertension Specialist from the European Society of Hypertension in 2020, recognized as a Diabetes Specialist in 2022, and received Emergency Medicine Specialization in 2023. She is currently working within the Emergency Department of AHEPA University Hospital of Thessaloniki, Aristotle University of Thessaloniki, Greece. Eleni teaches undergraduate and postgraduate students of the Medical School of Aristotle University of Thessaloniki. She has participated in more than 25 scientific projects, as a coordinator of 5 of these, and published her scientific work in various books and journals (more than 90). Eleni has participated as an invited lecturer or coordinator in various conferences (international and national) and received 12 awards (3 international) in recognition of her scientific work and its impact.

Journal of Personalized Medicine

MDPI

Article

Increased Complement Activation and Decreased ADAMTS13 Activity Are Associated with Genetic Susceptibility in Patients with Preeclampsia/HELLP Syndrome Compared to Healthy Pregnancies: An Observational Case-Controlled Study

Theodora-Maria Venou [1,†], Evangelia Vetsiou [1,†], Christos Varelas [2], Angelos Daniilidis [3], Kyriakos Psarras [4], Evaggelia-Evdoxia Koravou [2], Maria Koutra [2], Tasoula Touloumenidou [2], Vasilis Tsolakidis [1], Apostolia Papalexandri [2], Fani Minti [5], Evdokia Mandala [6], Konstantinos Dinas [7], Efthymia Vlachaki [1,*] and Eleni Gavriilaki [8]

1 Hematological Laboratory, 2nd Department of Internal Medicine, Aristotle University of Thessaloniki, Hippokration General Hospital, 54642 Thessaloniki, Greece; evangelia.vetsiou1@nhs.net (E.V.); v_tsolakidis@hotmail.com (V.T.)

2 Hematology Department, Papanicolaou General Hospital, 57010 Thessaloniki, Greece; cvarelas@auth.gr (C.V.); evakikor@gmail.com (E.-E.K.); tmdmgr@gmail.com (M.K.); tasoulatouloumenidou@gmail.com (T.T.); molbiol.gpapanikolaou@n3syzefxis.gov (A.P.)

3 1st Department of Obstetrics and Gynecology, Aristotle University of Thessaloniki, Papageorgiou General Hospital, 56429 Thessaloniki, Greece; angedan@auth.gr

4 2nd Propedeutical Department of Surgery, Aristotle University of Thessaloniki, Hippokration General Hospital, 54642 Thessaloniki, Greece; psarrask@auth.gr

5 Department of Medicine, School of Health Sciences, Aristotle University of Thessaloniki, 54124 Thessaloniki, Greece; fani.minti@yahoo.com

6 4th Department of Internal Medicine, Aristotle University of Thessaloniki, Hippokration General Hospital, 54642 Thessaloniki, Greece; emandala@auth.gr

7 2nd Department of Obstetrics and Gynecology, Aristotle University of Thessaloniki, Hippokration General Hospital, 54642 Thessaloniki, Greece

8 2nd Propedeutical Department of Internal Medicine, Aristotle University of Thessaloniki, Hippokration General Hospital, 54642 Thessaloniki, Greece; gavriiel@auth.gr

* Correspondence: efivlachaki@auth.gr

† These authors contributed equally to this work.

Abstract: Preeclampsia is a progressive multi-systemic disorder characterized by proteinuria, critical organ damage, and new-onset hypertension. It can be further complicated by HELLP syndrome (hemolysis, elevated liver enzymes, low platelets), resulting in critical liver or renal damage, disseminated coagulation, and grand mal seizures. This study aimed to examine the involvement of ADAMTS13, von Willebrand, and the complement system in the pathogenesis of preeclampsia/HELLP syndrome. We studied 30 Caucasian preeclamptic pregnant women and a control group of 15 healthy pregnancies. Genetic sequencing of ADAMTS13 and complement regulatory genes (MiniSeq System, Illumina) was performed. The modified Ham test was used to check for complement activation, ADAMTS13 activity, von Willebrand antigen (vWFAg) levels, and soluble C5b-9 levels were measured. Patients with preeclampsia had a decreased ADAMTS13 activity and increased C5b-9 levels. The vWFAg was significantly correlated with ADAMTS13 activity ($r = 0.497$, $p = 0.003$). Risk-factor variants were found in the genes of ADAMTS13, C3, thrombomodulin, CFB, CFH, MBL2, and, finally, MASP2. A portion of pregnant women with preeclampsia showed a decline in ADAMTS13 activity, correlated with vWFAg levels. These patients also exhibited an elevated complement activation and high-risk genetic variants in regulatory genes. Further research is needed to determine if these factors can serve as reliable biomarkers.

Keywords: preeclampsia; HELLP syndrome; pregnancy-associated liver disease; ADAMTS13; complement system; next-generation sequencing; C5b-9

1. Introduction

Preeclampsia (PE) is a common pregnancy-specific disorder with high mortality and morbidity rates worldwide. As a clinical entity belonging to the broad group of hypertensive disorders of pregnancy, it is defined as new-onset hypertension combined with proteinuria or other final-stage organ damage after 20 weeks of gestation [1]. This health condition is also classified under the umbrella of pregnancy-related liver disorders and can be further complicated by HELLP syndrome (hemolysis, elevated liver enzymes, low platelets), resulting in critical liver or renal damage, disseminated coagulation, and the development of grand mal seizures (eclampsia) [2].

PE understanding has seen major advances over the last twenty years; however, the exact pathophysiologic mechanisms still need to be determined. Until today, placental maternal vascular and metabolic malfunctions have been identified as crucial factors in its pathogenesis. Several processes, such as mutations; endothelial and trophoblast dysfunction, including spiral artery remodeling, low oxygenation of the placenta, and oxidative stress; impairment of the immunotolerance at the maternal–fetal surface; and an imbalance among angiogenic and antiangiogenic factors, have been implicated as contributing factors [1,2]. Establishing new reliable biomarkers in diagnosing PE/HELLP syndrome is of unparalleled importance for the earliest possible diagnosis and treatment.

Among immune mechanisms, there is piling interest in the involvement of the complement system and its overactivation in PE. Under normal circumstances, the complement system, an innate defense mechanism, is suppressed during pregnancy, sustaining the maternal immunological tolerance and allowing the successful development of the fetus [3]. Sparse studies suggest that the complement pathways elude the regulating suppressing mechanisms and promote inflammation through augmented terminal activation, further damaging the utero–placenta unit and disrupting the placenta perfusion [3,4]. The terminal complement component C5b-9 (membrane attack complex) is commonly detected in urine and placental samples of preeclamptic women, while other earlier complement components are also identified in patient samples, indicating the participation of the complement cascade in the pathogenesis of PE [2,4,5].

Several studies have linked PE and HELLP to dysregulated hemostasis and thrombotic microangiopathies (TMAs), which are characterized by elevated levels of the von Willebrand factor antigen (vWFAg) and reduced plasma activity of ADAMTS13 (a disintegrin and metalloproteinase with a thrombospondin type 1 motif, member 13) [2,6]. Over the last decade, significant progress has been made in developing clinical and laboratory approaches to predict disease course and genotype–phenotype correlations. It has been reported that, in patients with TMAs, ADAMTS13 single nucleotide polymorphisms (SNPs) can lead to partial deficiency when a primary trigger is present or when a mutation in a complement gene is co-inherited, indicating that, except for the clinical characteristics, the implicated pathophysiological mechanisms are also similar [7].

The use of ADAMTS13 activity is important for patients diagnosed with preeclampsia for several reasons. Preeclampsia/HELLP syndrome shares clinical features with thrombotic microangiopathies (TMAs) such as thrombotic thrombocytopenic purpura (TTP) and hemolytic–uremic syndrome (HUS). The measurement of ADAMTS13 activity can help differentiate between these conditions. In TTP, there is a typically severe ADAMTS13 deficiency, leading to excessive von Willebrand factor activity and microthrombi formation, while in preeclampsia, ADAMTS13 activity is usually lower but within normal range. Nevertheless, investigating ADAMTS13 activity in preeclampsia can provide insights into the underlying pathophysiological mechanisms of the disorder. Dysregulation of the balance between vWF and ADAMTS13 has been implicated in endothelial dysfunction and thrombotic microangiopathy, which are central features of preeclampsia. In summary, measuring the ADAMTS13 activity in patients diagnosed with preeclampsia is important for accurate diagnosis, prognostication, guiding therapeutic decisions, and advancing our understanding of the pathophysiology of this complex disorder [1].

Our research is grounded in the hypothesis that additional factors beyond the established ones may contribute to the development of preeclampsia (PE) and HELLP syndrome. To explore this hypothesis, our study aims to investigate the potential involvement of ADAMTS13, von Willebrand factor, and the complement system in the pathogenesis of these conditions. Preeclampsia is a complex disorder with multifactorial origins and, while certain mechanisms have been identified, there remains a need to uncover novel pathways that could elucidate its etiology and improve clinical management. Therefore, our research endeavors to delve into the roles of ADAMTS13 and the complement system, both of which have been implicated in endothelial dysfunction and thrombotic microangiopathy, key features of PE and HELLP syndrome. Additionally, we seek to explore how variations in the genes associated with ADAMTS13 and the complement system might impact the occurrence and severity of these pregnancy complications. By investigating these potential contributors, we aim to expand our understanding of the pathophysiology of PE and HELLP syndrome, potentially paving the way for novel diagnostic and therapeutic strategies to improve maternal and fetal outcomes.

2. Materials and Methods

2.1. Study Population

We conducted an observational, case–control study examining pregnant women with early onset severe preeclampsia and healthy pregnant women with similar age and gestational weeks. All participants provided written consent after receiving comprehensive information about the study's purpose and process. The study was conducted according to the guidelines of the Declaration of Helsinki and was approved by the Aristotle University of Thessaloniki Research Ethics Committee (protocol number: 22/5-2-2019).

Antenatal recruitment of pregnant women from the Department of Obstetrics and Gynecology of Hippokration General Hospital of Thessaloniki was conducted between July 2019 and March 2021. The diagnosis of preeclampsia was made in accordance with the American College of Obstetricians and Gynecologists criteria, which stipulates that a single incidence of systolic blood pressure (SBP) > 160; or diastolic blood pressure (DBP) > 110; or two instances of SBP > 140 or DBP > 90 with proteinuria or evidence of end-organ damage should be present [8]. Patients with pre-existing hypertensive conditions or a history of preeclampsia, HELLP syndrome, blood type O, antiphospholipid syndrome, or other autoimmune disorders and complement-mediated disease were excluded from the study. Medical records provided clinical variables such as systolic and diastolic blood pressure, as well as clinical laboratory parameters including random sample urine protein, serum creatinine, platelets, hemoglobin, glutamic-oxaloacetic transaminase (SGOT), glutamic-pyruvic transferase (SGPT), total bilirubin, and lactate dehydrogenase (LDH).

2.2. Laboratory Analysis

Peripheral blood and urine samples were collected on the day of enrolment. We performed genetic sequencing of the ADAMTS13 gene, as well as other complement regulatory genes (Complement factor H/CFH, CFH-related, CFI, CFB, CFD, C3, CD55, C5, MCP, thrombomodulin/THBD, MASP1, MASP2, MBL2, COLEC11, FCN1, and FCN3) with the use of Illumina MiniSeq sequencing System. DNA extraction from peripheral blood mononuclear was performed according to the Qiagen protocol.

The Modified Ham (mHam) test was utilized as an in vitro functional assay to evaluate complement activation. The mHam assay quantifies complement activation as a percentage of complement-mediated cell death, making it a functional assay. The testing process involves plating PIGA-null TF-1 cells into 96-well plates that contain gelatin veronal buffer with calcium and magnesium (GVB11; B102; Complement Technology Inc., Tyler, TX, USA). Subsequently, the cells are incubated at 37 °C for 15 min with diluted patient serum (1:5). After that, the cells are incubated at 37 °C for 2 h with diluted (1:10) WST-1 proliferation reagent (Roche, Basel, Switzerland). The absorbance is measured at 450 nm with a 630 nm filter in an ELISA plate reader (iMark Microplate Absorbance Reader, Biorad, Hercules,

CA, USA). Using the sample's absorbance and the heat-inactivated control's absorbance, the percentage of non-viable cells is calculated to determine complement activation. The samples are tested in triplicates.

The ADAMTS13 activity and soluble C5b-9 levels were quantified using commercially available ELISA (enzyme-linked immunosorbent assay, iMark Microplate Absorbance Reader, Biorad) kits (Quidel, San Diego, CA, USA), following the manufacturer's instructions. The measurement of vWFAg was carried out utilizing the immunoturbidimetric assay with the Siemens Healthineers BCS® XP System. The ratios of vWFAg to ADAMTS13 activity (vWFAg/ADAMTS13) and platelets count to mean platelet volume (PLTs/MPV) were also calculated.

2.3. Bioinformatics and Statistical Analysis

The Statistical Package for Social Sciences (SPSS 27.0.1.0) statistical program for windows version 27 was used to perform statistical analysis in this study. Due to the small sample size and non-normal distribution of the investigated parameters, we utilized the non-parametric Mann–Whitney test to compare the two independent groups. Additionally, we performed Levene's test to assess the equality of variances. The relationship between mHam test results and preeclampsia occurrence was discovered using the Chi-squared test. The level of statistical significance was set to 0.05. The median value and interquartile range of each parameter were calculated by group. Furthermore, a post hoc power analysis was conducted, which confirmed that the study population was adequate for a significance level of 5% and the desired power level of 80%.

To establish the clinical significance of the detected genetic variants, four bioinformatic tools (SIFT, PolyPhen-2, PROVEAN, and CADD) were used. It is worth mentioning that we considered every variant which was characterized as damaging by 2 or more bioinformatic tools as deleterious.

3. Results

3.1. Study Population

Table 1 presents the baseline characteristics of the two study groups. The patients' group included 30 Caucasian preeclamptic pregnant women with a median age of 36 years [median age (IQR): 36 (10, 29–39)] and a median gestational age of 32 weeks. The control group, on the other hand, comprised 15 healthy pregnant women with a median age of 30 years [median age (IQR): 30 (11, 27–38) years] and a median gestational age of 30 weeks. Both groups shared similar baseline characteristics, and the control group had otherwise uncomplicated pregnancies.

Table 1. Baseline characteristics and laboratory tests of the study population [median (interquartile range—IQR)], level of statistical significance: 0.05 (Mann—Whitney test).

	Preeclamptic Group	Healthy Control Group	p
Age (years)	36 [10 (29–39)]	30 [11 (27–38)]	0.22
Gestational week	32 [3 (31–34)]	30 [9 (25–34)]	0.07
Hb (g/dL)	11.9 [2.1 (11.1–13.2)]	10.4 [2.4 (9.2–11.6)]	0.01
PLTs (/mm^3)	219.000 [74.000 (187.500–261.500)]	253.000 [66.250 (206.500–272.750)]	0.60
SGOT (IU/L)	17.5 [10 (15–25)]	14 [4 (11–15)]	0.003
SGPT (IU/L)	16 [11 (12–23)]	11 [7 (8.25–15.25)]	0.72
Total bilirubin (mg/dL)	0.33 [0.18 (0.22–0.4)]	0.37 [0.12 (0.32–0.44)]	0.12
Serum Creatine (mg/dL)	0.71 [0.26 (0.62–0.88)]	0.67 [0.12 (0.6–0.72)]	0.029
Serum LDH (units/L)	191 [47 (175–222)]	190 [66 (160–226)]	0.43

Table 1. *Cont.*

	Preeclamptic Group	Healthy Control Group	p
Urine protein (mg)	129 [280 (18–298)]	0	0.025
Systolic Blood Pressure (mmHg)	165 [27 (150–177]	124 [13 (116–129)]	<0.001
Diastolic Blood Pressure (mmHg)	100 [20 (90–110)]	82 [11 (76–87)]	<0.001

Hb: Hemoglobin, PLTs: platelets, SGOT: serum glutamic-oxaloacetic transaminase, SGPT: serum-glutamic pyruvic transaminase, LDH: lactate dehydrogenase.

The results of the study revealed a noteworthy disparity between the subjects with preeclampsia and the control group. Specifically, individuals with preeclampsia demonstrated a higher level of serum creatine and urine protein, with a statistically significant difference ($p = 0.029$ and $p = 0.025$, respectively). Additionally, a statistically significant difference was observed between the two groups concerning hemoglobin ($p = 0.01$), with the healthy control group displaying a lower median value. This notable difference could potentially be attributed to inadequate plasma expansion.

When it comes to liver function tests, it has been discovered that women who suffer from preeclampsia have significantly higher SGOT serum levels compared to healthy individuals in the control group ($p = 0.003$). However, there seems to be no significant difference in the levels of serum SGPT or total bilirubin between the two groups ($p = 0.72$ and $p = 0.12$, respectively). It is worth mentioning that none of the women in either group had elevated levels of serum total bilirubin. All participants in the healthy control group exhibited normal liver function test results. However, in the group of women with preeclampsia, three individuals showed elevated levels of SGOT, SGPT, or both, but none of them had a positive mHam test or increased C5b-9 levels.

Furthermore, it was interesting to find that ADAMTS13 activity was significantly lower in patients with preeclampsia [median (IQR, p25–p75): 70.1% (16.9, 65.3–82.2) vs. 89.5% (25.2, 71.8–97), $p = 0.012$], but remained within normal limits in both groups. Meanwhile, the levels of soluble C5b-9, as a biomarker of terminal complement activation, were increased in the group of patients with preeclampsia when compared to the healthy control [median (IQR, p25–p75): 311 ng/mL (386, 7–394) versus 35 ng/mL (5.2, 31–36.2)]. The difference was statistically significant between the two groups ($p = 0.007$). In addition, the modified HAM test was positive only in preeclamptic women (11/30, 36%) ($p = 0.008$). It is worth noting that all the patients in the preeclamptic group who tested positive for the mHam test also had elevated C5b-9 levels, indicating increased complement activation in this group of patients.

Moreover, the vWFAg was significantly correlated with ADAMTS13 activity ($r = 0.497$, $p = 0.003$). However, no statistically significant difference was observed between the two groups in terms of the vWFAg/ADAMTS13 ratio ($p > 0.05$). Furthermore, there was no statistically significant difference found between the two groups concerning the ratio of PLTs/MPV (p: 0.33 > 0.05). This ratio is expected to be lower in those with preeclampsia, as compared to healthy pregnant women due to a decline in PLTs count and an increase in MPV. Finally, no significant association was found between liver function tests (SGOT, SGPT, and total bilirubin) and C5b-9 levels or ADAMTS13 activity ($p > 0.05$).

3.2. Genetic Analysis

Conducting an initial evaluation to detect clinically significant variations by utilizing the ClinVar annotated data (analysis A), risk-factor variants were detected in the genes of ADAMTS13 (rs2301612), C3 (rs2230199), and Complement Factor H, CFH (rs800292). The finding of double heterozygosity in these genes was exclusive to preeclamptic women and, more specifically, to approximately half of them (16/30, 54%, $p < 0.001$). It is worth noting that, among the entire group of women with preeclampsia, only one individual exhibited indications of renal injury, as evidenced by a serum creatinine level of 1.51 g/dL and an estimated glomerular filtration rate (eGFR) of 43 mL/min per 1.73 m^2, calculated using the MDRD equation: 175 × SerumCr-1.154 × age − 0.203 × 1.212 (if patient is black) × 0.742 (if female). This pregnant woman tested positive for the modified Ham test (C5b-9: 1232 ng/mL, ADAMTS13: 31%), and possessed double heterozygosity for high-risk genetic variants. Moreover, it should be mentioned that that there was an individual with preeclampsia who had a marked increase in liver enzyme levels (SGOT = 982 IU/L and SGPT = 1151 IU/L), but the mHAM test came back negative and normal C5b-9 serum levels were detected (C5b-9 = 49.2 ng/mL). In the preeclamptic pregnant woman with abnormal liver function tests, no high-risk genetic variants were identified.

Afterward, a further analysis was performed (analysis B) with the use of four bioinformatic tools and five deleterious genetic variants were identified in seven pregnant women suffering from preeclampsia. However, the same genetic variants were found only in three pregnant women in the healthy control group. The identified genetic variants are associated with the gene of ADAMTS13 (rs28503257 and rs28647808), thrombomodulin (rs1800579), CFB (rs12614), CFH (rs35274867), MBL2 (rs503073, rs1800450, and rs1800451), and finally MASP2 (rs12711521, rs139962539, and rs72550870).

As per the study, patients who had clinically significant variants that were identified in both analysis A and analysis B (in the ADAMTS13, thrombomodulin, CFB, CFH, MBL2, MASP2, and C3 genes) showed a significant decrease in vWFAg levels compared to those who did not have such variants (177 vs. 295, $p = 0.004$). Conversely, patients with the rs1800450 variant in the lectin gene showed a significant increase in vWFAg levels (276 vs. 30, $p = 0.038$).

4. Discussion

The present non-interventional, case–control study supports the findings of other research groups. The study reveals a statistically significant reduction in ADAMTS13 activity and an elevation in soluble C5b-9 levels among a group of pregnant women who developed early onset severe preeclampsia, compared to a healthy control group. Furthermore, the investigation identified a number of genetic variants in the genes of ADAMTS13, C3, CFH, CFB, thrombomodulin, MBL2, and MASP2 that were significantly linked with the occurrence of preeclampsia, according to the results of analyses A and B.

It has been a commonly held belief that the primary pathophysiological mechanism of preeclampsia is angiogenic imbalance, until recent times [3]. Endothelial cells and megakaryocytes are responsible for producing a complex glycoprotein called von Willebrand factor (vWF) in the form of preproprotein ultra large VWF (ULVWF). The ULVWF multimers are subsequently cleaved into less reactive vWF dimers and eliminated from circulation by ADAMTS13, which acts as its exclusive substrate. [6]. ADAMTS13's involvement in the pathophysiology of PE/HELLP syndrome remains elusive. However, the common clinical presentation of TMAs, such as thrombotic thrombocytopenic purpura (TTP), in which ADAMTS13's role is well understood [9,10], and PE/HELLP syndrome, suggests a linkage between the faulted expression of ADAMTS13 and the development of PE/HELLP syndrome [11].

An ADAMTS13 activity level of less than 10% is a strong indication of TTP diagnosis in relevant clinical contexts. However, several medical facilities lack the necessary equipment to perform the test on-site, necessitating the sending of samples to a reference laboratory, which further delays diagnosis. The differentiation between TTP and preeclampsia/HELLP syndrome is frequently based on coexisting clinical parameters. It is critical to distinguish between these two clinical entities, due to the contrasting management options. Delivery is the preferred treatment option for preeclampsia and the condition typically resolves within a few days after delivery. Nevertheless, delivery is not an appropriate treatment for TTP because symptoms continue to progress postpartum without plasmapheresis [12].

There is a question as to whether ADAMTS13 can be used as a reliable biomarker to diagnose preeclampsia/HELLP syndrome. In accordance with our findings, several studies found statistically significant decreases in ADAMTS13 activity in preeclamptic women's serums over healthy controls [6,11,13–17]. A few articles, however, found no significant differences between the two groups of individuals, suggesting that ADAMTS13 activity is not associated with PE [18–20]. Consequently, besides the strong correlation between significantly low levels of ADAMTS13 activity (below 10–20%) and TTP, a more average level cannot rule out preeclampsia. However, the absence of ADAMTS13 activity cannot be equated with a diagnosis of preeclampsia [21].

Interestingly, in agreement with the results of our study, increasing evidence suggests that the terminal complement proteins C5a and C5b-9 are also involved in the pathogenesis of preeclampsia. Studies have suggested that PE is ultimately a complement-mediated disease, with the complement system being fundamental to its inflammatory process. The circulation of PE patients has been found to contain elevated amounts of complement components and their activation derivatives, such as C5a and C5b-9 complexes, even though the data are highly contradictory in this area [22]. It was also found that preeclamptic women's trophoblasts accumulated more C5b-9 than non-preeclamptic women [23]. Moreover, in the study of Youssef et al., significantly higher levels of C5b-9 were detected in endothelial cells exposed to the plasma of pregnant women with severe preeclampsia at an early stage of pregnancy [5].

In a similar manner to our study, the involvement of the complement system in the hemolysis of severe PE was showcased in the study of Vaught et al., in which the complement activity was identified through a modified Ham test in ex vivo experiments [24]. It should be mentioned that the mHam test has been used as an indicator of complement system activation in other complement-mediated conditions, such as uremic hemolytic syndrome (aHUS) [25]. In another study, most patients with a diagnosis of HELLP had a positive mHam test (62%) compared to the healthy control group (16%), with a statistically significant difference between the two groups ($p < 0.001$). The results were similar in the group of patients with aHUS (88% versus 16%, $p < 0.001$) [26]. Therefore, even if a positive mHam test is not indicative of preeclampsia, the possibility of a complement system role in preeclampsia pathogenesis is highly plausible.

Moreover, the study of Burwick et al. demonstrated that there was no statistically significant difference between pregnant women with preeclampsia and pregnant women with chronic hypertension regarding plasma levels of C5b-9. This finding makes it unclear whether increased levels of plasma C5b-9 are specific to preeclampsia or merely suggest an increased risk of developing a number of clinical entities within the general category of hypertensive disorders of pregnancy. As part of the same study, C5b-9 excretion in urine was found to be a highly reliable biomarker for discriminating between severe preeclampsia and chronic hypertension in two different groups of pregnant women [27].

Liver disorders that may occur during pregnancy are unique and require special attention. There are several clinical conditions that can cause abnormal liver function tests during pregnancy, including hyperemesis gravidarum, intrahepatic cholestasis of pregnancy, acute fatty liver of pregnancy, and preeclampsia/HELLP syndrome [28]. It is important to keep in mind that pregnant women who have severe preeclampsia may encounter liver enzyme abnormalities, affecting up to 10% of cases. These abnormalities are usually identified by the presence of two to three times more alanine and aspartate aminotransferases than normal [29].

A study carried out by Valencia et al. showed significantly low plasma and high urine C5b-9 levels, which were correlated with end-organ damage in a group of pregnant women suffering from severe preeclampsia. It is possible that preeclampsia is caused by complement-mediated end-organ damage, as evidenced by the decreased plasma levels of complement system components combined with their increased excretion in urine. The same study found that hypertensive pregnant women without signs of organ dysfunction or other laboratory abnormalities did not exhibit a significant decrease in plasma C5b-9 levels [30]. We identified one woman who had signs of renal damage (increased creatinine and decreased eGFR) and high plasma levels of C5b-9 (C5b-9: 1232 ng/mL). In our study, no other individual in the preeclamptic group showed any signs of end-organ damage and this is possibly the reason why significantly increased levels of C5b-9 were measured in their plasma compared to the control group.

Overall, according to the available research, complement control is disrupted in many women who develop preeclampsia and HELLP syndrome, and terminal complement activation is enhanced. These data imply that inhibiting the terminal complement pathway constitutes a promising field of investigation for new drug development in the future. In the literature, eculizumab, a C5 inhibitor, has been shown to be effective in treating severe preeclampsia, reducing the production of C5a. Pregnant women and fetuses are not believed to be at risk from eculizumab treatment [31,32].

Using next-generation sequencing (NGS), large genomic regions can be analyzed, allowing new possibilities to emerge. However, NGS has been slowly adopted for research on female reproductive health [33]. Based on the current knowledge of PE pathology, candidate gene studies have compared the genetic variation frequency among patients and controls to identify potential associations, such as the genes involved in endothelial function and blood pressure regulation (VEFGR-1, TGF-β, Eng, RAS, AGT, ACE, AGTR1, and eNOS), genes associated with lipid metabolism and oxidative stress (EPHX1, GST, NOX1, SOD2, APOE, LPL, and ROS), as well as thrombophilic genes (F5, F2, and MTHFR) [34]. In our study, risk-factor variants were found in ADAMTD13, C3, and Complement Factor H (CFH) genes. It is worth noting that the study conducted by von Krogh et al. did not find any correlation between the three investigated gene variants of ADAMTS13 and PE, including the rs28647808 variant, which our own study characterized as deleterious [20].

According to Lokki et al., the function of C3 can be affected due to variants in crucial domains of the C3 gene, simultaneously associated with the severity of the disease. Variant rs2230199 in C3 is known as the slow/fast mutation affecting the mobility of the protein during the electrophoresis process and was associated with the pathogenesis of PE [35]. On the other hand, other published studies found no correlation between this specific variant and preeclampsia [36,37]. Interestingly, according to Banadakoppa et al., the high-risk variant rs800292 in the CFH gene is associated with the activation of the alternative pathway in patients with preeclampsia, only in the coexistence of a variant in the CD46 gene [38].

A key strength of the present study is the use of standard laboratory techniques, such as ELISA, for measuring ADAMTS13 activity and C5b-9 activity, which could facilitate their establishment as biomarkers. A simple process, mHam, can also easily be incorporated into clinical practice in various complement-mediated diseases as an indicator of the activation of the complement system.

The present study has some limitations worth mentioning. As a starting point, a larger sample size is necessary to increase the power of the study and reach valid conclusions. Collecting a larger sample can be challenging, especially for pregnant women with a preeclampsia diagnosis, since appropriate treatment might be required immediately. Due to the small sample size and the variability of illness in severe preeclamptic women, our conclusions are limited. The findings of this study cannot be generalized to women with mild preeclampsia or those with atypical disease. As a result of our findings, we can support the hypothesis that active disease in severe preeclampsia is typically associated with a dysregulation of the complement system. Nevertheless, in order to establish that complement indicators may indicate illness onset, additional research is required.

Finally, "Next Generation Sequencing" is a relatively new technology that has not been widely adopted, requiring specialized equipment and qualified personnel that are not always available. As a matter of fact, organizing a larger cohort is a difficult but significant undertaking. A further limitation of the present study is that only C5b-9 serum levels were measured. C5b-9 is part of the common pathway of complement activation. Therefore, we could not investigate which of the pathways (classical, lectin, or alternative) ultimately activates the complement system.

5. Conclusions

The results of our study indicate that a specific group of pregnant women suffering from preeclampsia demonstrated a decline in ADAMTS13 activity, which exhibited a positive correlation with vWFAg levels. These findings point towards potential endothelial damage and may warrant further investigation. Additionally, a subset of patients diagnosed with preeclampsia exhibit escalated complement activation, along with the presence of high-risk genetic variants in regulatory genes. Further research is required to determine whether these factors could potentially serve as dependable biomarkers for predicting the course of the disease, aiding in diagnosis, or even as promising therapeutic agents.

Author Contributions: T.-M.V.: methodology, validation, formal analysis, investigation, resources, data curation, writing, E.V. (Evangelia Vetsiou): methodology, validation, formal analysis, investigation, resources, data curation, writing, C.V.: methodology, validation, formal analysis, investigation, resources, data curation, writing, A.D.: formal analysis, investigation, resources, K.P.: formal analysis, investigation, resources, E.-E.K.: formal analysis, investigation, resources, M.K.: formal analysis, investigation, resources, T.T.: formal analysis, investigation, resources, V.T.: formal analysis, investigation, resources, A.P.: formal analysis, investigation, resources, F.M.: formal analysis, investigation, resources, E.M.: formal analysis, investigation, resources, K.D.: formal analysis, investigation, resources, E.V. (Efthymia Vlachaki): conceptualization, methodology, validation, formal analysis, investigation, resources, data curation, writing, visualization, supervision, project administration, E.G.: conceptualization, methodology, validation, formal analysis, investigation, resources, data curation, writing, visualization, supervision, project administration. All authors have read and agreed to the published version of the manuscript.

Funding: This research received no external funding.

Institutional Review Board Statement: This study was conducted according to the guidelines of the Declaration of Helsinki and was approved by the Aristotle University of Thessaloniki Research Ethics Committee (protocol number: 22/5-2-2019).

Informed Consent Statement: Informed consent was obtained from all subjects involved in the study.

Data Availability Statement: The data presented in this study are not available due to ethical reasons.

Conflicts of Interest: The authors declare no conflicts of interest.

References

1. Gardikioti, A.; Venou, T.-M.; Gavriilaki, E.; Vetsiou, E.; Mavrikou, I.; Dinas, K.; Daniilidis, A.; Vlachaki, E. Molecular Advances in Preeclampsia and HELLP Syndrome. *Int. J. Mol. Sci.* **2022**, *23*, 3851. [CrossRef] [PubMed]
2. Phipps, E.A.; Thadhani, R.; Benzing, T.; Karumanchi, S.A. Pre-Eclampsia: Pathogenesis, Novel Diagnostics and Therapies. *Nat. Rev. Nephrol.* **2019**, *15*, 275–289. [CrossRef] [PubMed]
3. Aneman, I.; Pienaar, D.; Suvakov, S.; Simic, T.P.; Garovic, V.D.; McClements, L. Mechanisms of Key Innate Immune Cells in Early- and Late-Onset Preeclampsia. *Front. Immunol.* **2020**, *11*, 567532. [CrossRef] [PubMed]
4. Regal, J.F.; Burwick, R.M.; Fleming, S.D. The Complement System and Preeclampsia. *Curr. Hypertens. Rep.* **2017**, *19*, 87. [CrossRef] [PubMed]
5. Youssef, L.; Miranda, J.; Blasco, M.; Paules, C.; Crovetto, F.; Palomo, M.; Torramade-Moix, S.; García-Calderó, H.; Tura-Ceide, O.; Dantas, A.P.; et al. Complement and Coagulation Cascades Activation Is the Main Pathophysiological Pathway in Early-Onset Severe Preeclampsia Revealed by Maternal Proteomics. *Sci. Rep.* **2021**, *11*, 3048. [CrossRef]
6. Alpoim, P.N.; Gomes, K.B.; Godoi, L.C.; Rios, D.R.; Carvalho, M.G.; Fernandes, A.P.; Dusse, L.M. ADAMTS13, FVIII, von Willebrand Factor, ABO Blood Group Assessment in Preeclampsia. *Clin. Chim. Acta* **2011**, *412*, 2162–2166. [CrossRef] [PubMed]
7. Fidalgo, T.; Martinho, P.; Pinto, C.S.; Oliveira, A.C.; Salvado, R.; Borràs, N.; Coucelo, M.; Manco, L.; Maia, T.; Mendes, M.J.; et al. Combined Study of ADAMTS13 and Complement Genes in the Diagnosis of Thrombotic Microangiopathies Using Next-Generation Sequencing. *Res. Pr. Thromb. Haemost.* **2017**, *1*, 69–80. [CrossRef] [PubMed]
8. Kallela, J.; Jääskeläinen, T.; Kortelainen, E.; Heinonen, S.; Kajantie, E.; Kere, J.; Kivinen, K.; Pouta, A.; Laivuori, H. The Diagnosis of Pre-Eclampsia Using Two Revised Classifications in the Finnish Pre-Eclampsia Consortium (FINNPEC) Cohort. *BMC Pregnancy Childbirth* **2016**, *16*, 221. [CrossRef] [PubMed]
9. Gupta, M.; Feinberg, B.B.; Burwick, R.M. Thrombotic Microangiopathies of Pregnancy: Differential Diagnosis. *Pregnancy Hypertens.* **2018**, *12*, 29–34. [CrossRef]
10. Zander, C.B.; Cao, W.; Zheng, X.L. ADAMTS13 and von Willebrand Factor Interactions. *Curr. Opin. Hematol.* **2015**, *22*, 452–459. [CrossRef]

11. Aref, S.; Goda, H. Increased VWF Antigen Levels and Decreased ADAMTS13 Activity in Preeclampsia. *Hematology* **2013**, *18*, 237–241. [CrossRef] [PubMed]
12. Pourrat, O.; Coudroy, R.; Pierre, F. Differentiation between Severe HELLP Syndrome and Thrombotic Microangiopathy, Thrombotic Thrombocytopenic Purpura and Other Imitators. *Eur. J. Obstet. Gynecol. Reprod. Biol.* **2015**, *189*, 68–72. [CrossRef] [PubMed]
13. Hulstein, J.J.J.; Van Runnard Heimel, P.J.; Franx, A.; Lenting, P.J.; Bruinse, H.W.; Silence, K.; De Groot, P.H.G.; Fijnheer, R. Acute Activation of the Endothelium Results in Increased Levels of Active von Willebrand Factor in Hemolysis, Elevated Liver Enzymes and Low Platelets (HELLP) Syndrome. *J. Thromb. Haemost.* **2006**, *4*, 2569–2575. [CrossRef] [PubMed]
14. Namlı Kalem, M.; Kalem, Z.; Yüce, T.; Soylemez, F. ADAMTS 1, 4, 12, and 13 Levels in Maternal Blood, Cord Blood, and Placenta in Preeclampsia. *Hypertens. Pregnancy* **2018**, *37*, 9–17. [CrossRef] [PubMed]
15. Stepanian, A.; Cohen-Moatti, M.; Sanglier, T.; Legendre, P.; Ameziane, N.; Tsatsaris, V.; Mandelbrot, L.; De Prost, D.; Veyradier, A. Von Willebrand Factor and ADAMTS13: A Candidate Couple for Preeclampsia Pathophysiology. *Arterioscler. Thromb. Vasc. Biol.* **2011**, *31*, 1703–1709. [CrossRef] [PubMed]
16. Sabau, L.; Terriou, L.; Provot, F.; Fourrier, F.; Roumier, C.; Caron, C.; Susen, S.; Ducloy-Bouthors, A.S. Are There Any Additional Mechanisms for Haemolysis in HELLP Syndrome. *Thromb. Res.* **2016**, *142*, 40–43. [CrossRef]
17. Xiao, J.; Feng, Y.; Li, X.; Li, W.; Fan, L.; Liu, J.; Zeng, X.; Chen, K.; Chen, X.; Zhou, X.; et al. Expression of ADAMTS13 in Normal and Abnormal Placentae and Its Potential Role in Angiogenesis and Placenta Development. *Arter. Thromb. Vasc. Biol.* **2017**, *37*, 1748–1756. [CrossRef] [PubMed]
18. Molvarec, A.; Rigó, J.; Bõze, T.; Derzsy, Z.; Cervenak, L.; Makó, V.; Gombos, T.; Udvardy, M.L.; Hársfalvi, J.; Prohászka, Z. Increased Plasma von Willebrand Factor Antigen Levels but Normal von Willebrand Factor Cleaving Protease (ADAHTS13) Activity in Preeclampsia. *Thromb. Haemost.* **2009**, *101*, 305–311. [CrossRef]
19. Yoshida, Y.; Matsumoto, M.; Yagi, H.; Isonishi, A.; Sakai, K.; Hayakawa, M.; Hori, Y.; Sado, T.; Kobayashi, H.; Fujimura, Y. Severe Reduction of Free-Form ADAMTS13, Unbound to von Willebrand Factor, in Plasma of Patients with HELLP Syndrome. *Blood Adv.* **2017**, *1*, 1628–1631. [CrossRef]
20. Von Krogh, A.S.; Kremer Hovinga, J.A.; Romundstad, P.R.; Roten, L.T.; Lämmle, B.; Waage, A.; Quist-Paulsen, P. ADAMTS13 Gene Variants and Function in Women with Preeclampsia: A Population-Based Nested Case-Control Study from the HUNT Study. *Thromb. Res.* **2015**, *136*, 282–288. [CrossRef]
21. Mousseaux, C.; Joly, B.S.; Mohamadou, I.; Arrestier, R.; Hertig, A.; Rafat, C. Severe HELLP Syndrome Masquerading as Thrombocytopenic Thrombotic Purpura: A Case Report. *BMC Nephrol.* **2020**, *21*, 204. [CrossRef] [PubMed]
22. Agostinis, C.; Mangogna, A.; Balduit, A.; Aghamajidi, A.; Ricci, G.; Kishore, U.; Bulla, R. COVID-19, Pre-Eclampsia, and Complement System. *Front. Immunol.* **2021**, *12*, 775168. [CrossRef] [PubMed]
23. Rampersad, R.; Barton, A.; Sadovsky, Y.; Nelson, D.M. The C5b-9 Membrane Attack Complex of Complement Activation Localizes to Villous Trophoblast Injury In Vivo and Modulates Human Trophoblast Function In Vitro. *Placenta* **2008**, *29*, 855–861. [CrossRef] [PubMed]
24. Vaught, A.J.; Gavriilaki, E.; Hueppchen, N.; Blakemore, K.; Yuan, X.; Seifert, S.M.; York, S.; Brodsky, R.A. Direct Evidence of Complement Activation in HELLP Syndrome: A Link to Atypical Hemolytic Uremic Syndrome. *Exp. Hematol.* **2016**, *44*, 390–398. [CrossRef] [PubMed]
25. Gavriilaki, E.; Yuan, X.; Ye, Z.; Ambinder, A.J.; Shanbhag, S.P.; Streiff, M.B.; Kickler, T.S.; Moliterno, A.R.; Sperati, C.J.; Brodsky, R.A. Modified Ham Test for Atypical Hemolytic Uremic Syndrome. *Blood* **2015**, *125*, 3637–3646. [CrossRef] [PubMed]
26. Vaught, A.J.; Braunstein, E.M.; Jasem, J.; Yuan, X.; Makhlin, I.; Eloundou, S.; Baines, A.C.; Merrill, S.A.; Chaturvedi, S.; Blakemore, K.; et al. Germline Mutations in the Alternative Pathway of Complement Predispose to HELLP Syndrome. *JCI Insight* **2018**, *3*, e99128. [CrossRef] [PubMed]
27. Burwick, R.M.; Fichorova, R.N.; Dawood, H.Y.; Yamamoto, H.S.; Feinberg, B.B. Urinary Excretion of C5b-9 in Severe Preeclampsia Tipping the Balance of Complement Activation in Pregnancy. *Hypertension* **2013**, *62*, 1040–1045. [CrossRef] [PubMed]
28. Terrault, N.A.; Williamson, C. Pregnancy-Associated Liver Diseases. *Gastroenterology* **2022**, *163*, 97–117.e1. [CrossRef] [PubMed]
29. Hammoud, G.M.; Ibdah, J.A. Preeclampsia-Induced Liver Dysfunction, HELLP Syndrome, and Acute Fatty Liver of Pregnancy. *Clin. Liver Dis.* **2014**, *4*, 67–73. [CrossRef]
30. Valencia, C.M.; Hersh, A.R.; Burwick, R.M.; Velásquez, J.A.; Gutiérrez-Marin, J.; Edna, F.; Silva, J.L.; Trujillo-Otalvaro, J.; Vargas-Rodríguez, J.; Bernal, Y.; et al. Soluble Concentrations of the Terminal Complement Complex C5b-9 Correlate with End-Organ Injury in Preeclampsia. *Pregnancy Hypertens.* **2022**, *29*, 92–97. [CrossRef]
31. Elabd, H.; Elkholi, M.; Steinberg, L.; Acharya, A. Eculizumab, a Novel Potential Treatment for Acute Kidney Injury Associated with Preeclampsia/HELLP Syndrome. *BMJ Case Rep.* **2019**, *12*, e228709. [CrossRef]
32. Burwick, R.M.; Feinberg, B.B. Eculizumab for the Treatment of Preeclampsia/HELLP Syndrome. *Placenta* **2013**, *34*, 201–203. [CrossRef] [PubMed]
33. Laissue, P.; Vaiman, D. Exploring the Molecular Aetiology of Preeclampsia by Massive Parallel Sequencing of DNA. *Curr. Hypertens. Rep.* **2020**, *22*, 31. [CrossRef] [PubMed]
34. Parada-Niño, L.; Castillo-León, L.F.; Morel, A. Preeclampsia, Natural History, Genes, and MiRNAs Associated with the Syndrome. *J. Pregnancy* **2022**, *2022*, 3851225. [CrossRef] [PubMed]

35. Inkeri Lokki, A.; Kaartokallio, T.; Holmberg, V.; Onkamo, P.; Koskinen, L.L.E.; Saavalainen, P.; Heinonen, S.; Kajantie, E.; Kere, J.; Kivinen, K.; et al. Analysis of Complement C3 Gene Reveals Susceptibility to Severe Preeclampsia. *Front. Immunol.* **2017**, *8*, 257172. [CrossRef]
36. Rhim, M.S.; Meddeb, S.; Kaabia, O.; Jalloul, M.; Sakouhi, M.; Jrzad, B.B.H.; Felah, R. C3F Gene Mutation Is Involved in the Susceptibility to Pre-Eclampsia. *Arch. Gynecol. Obs.* **2015**, *291*, 1023–1027. [CrossRef] [PubMed]
37. Cooper, D.W.; Deane, E.M.; Marshall, P.; Galleryb, E.D.M. C3 Allotypes in Pregnancy Hypertension and Eclampsia. *Hum. Hered.* **1988**, *38*, 52–55. [CrossRef]
38. Banadakoppa, M.; Balakrishnan, M.; Yallampalli, C. Common Variants of Fetal and Maternal Complement Genes in Preeclampsia: Pregnancy Specific Complotype. *Sci. Rep.* **2020**, *10*, 4811. [CrossRef]

Journal of *Personalized Medicine*

MDPI

Article

The Hemodynamic Profile and Intraoperative Bleeding Impact on Liver Transplant Patients

Lavinia Nicoleta Brezeanu [1,*,†], Cosmina Elena Jercălău [2,†], Catalina Liliana Andrei [2], Octavian Ceban [3] and Gabriela Droc [1,4]

1 Department of Anaesthesia and Intensive Care I, Fundeni Clinical Institute, 022322 Bucharest, Romania; gabidroc@gmail.com
2 Department of Cardiology, "Bagdasar Arseni" Emergency Hospital, "Carol Davila" University of Medicine and Pharmacy, 050474 Bucharest, Romania; cosmina-elena.jercalau@drd.umfcd.ro (C.E.J.); catalina.andrei@umfcd.ro (C.L.A.)
3 Economic Cybernetics and Informatics Department, The Bucharest University of Economic Studies, 010374 Bucharest, Romania; octavianceban1995@gmail.com
4 Department of Anaesthesia and Intensive Care, "Carol Davila" University of Medicine and Pharmacy, 419291 Bucharest, Romania
* Correspondence: laviniajipa11@yahoo.com; Tel.: +40-723471034
† These authors contributed equally to this work.

Abstract: Liver transplantation is the treatment of choice for end-stage liver disease and despite accumulated experience over the years, improved surgical techniques, better immunosuppression and adequate intensive care management, it still represents the greatest challenge for anesthesiologists. The aim of the study was the characterization of the hemodynamic profile of patients with liver cirrhosis undergoing liver transplantation with the help of the PiCCO system during the three surgical stages, the impact of bleeding on hemodynamic status and correlation between the amount of bleeding, lactate levels, severity scores and survival rate and complications. Another focus of this study was the amount of transfused blood products and their impact on postoperative complications. Our study included 70 patients who underwent liver transplantation in our center and were hemodynamically monitored with the PiCCO system. Data were processed using the Python 3.9 programming language. Results: The mean MELD severity score was 18 points. During surgery, significant variations in the hemodynamic parameters occurred. All patients had a decrease in cardiac output in the anhepatic phase, with 50% presenting a decrease of more than 40%. In total, 78% of patients showed a decrease in the global ejection fraction, with a median value of 30%.Overall, 75% of patients had a total blood loss of less than 6000 mL and 31 patients developed immediate postoperative complications with a 50% probability with blood loss exceeding 6500 mL. Seven patients (10%) did not survive after 30 days. An amount of 5 mmol/L of serum neohepatic lactate determines a 50% probability of complications. Conclusions: Surgical technique causes an important decrease in cardiac output. Intraoperative bleeding has a major impact on outcome and the first month represents a critical period after liver transplantation. Statistical tests describe the probability of 30/90-day survival and the occurrence of complications according to variables such as intraoperative bleeding and MELD severity score. Intraoperative transfusion correlates with the occurrence of postoperative complications.

Keywords: liver transplantation; hemodynamic monitoring; PiCCO system; 30/90-day survival probabilities

1. Introduction

Liver transplantation is the treatment of choice for end-stage liver disease. Since the first successful liver transplant in 1967, the survival rate has improved considerably [1,2]. Despite numerous developments in surgical techniques, immunosuppression as well as perioperative anesthetic management, anesthesia for liver transplantation is considered the greatest challenge for anesthesiologists. It requires extensive experience as well as good knowledge of the pathophysiology of liver disease and its systemic manifestations. The cirrhotic patient is a high-risk patient with alterations in cardiovascular, pulmonary, hepatic and renal systems who also presents with coagulation disorders.

Cirrhotic patients usually present with a hyperdynamic status, with increased cardiac output and decreased systemic vascular resistance. Some patients present cirrhotic cardiomyopathy with impaired contractility and prolonged QT [3,4]. An early diagnosis of hemodynamic instability during liver transplantation as well as its prompt management are two of the most important factors for a favorable prognosis. Various modalities have emerged over time for adequate cardiac output monitoring [5]. The pulmonary artery catheter (Swan Ganz) was initially used, but studies have shown that it is no longer the gold standard for cardiac output monitoring in liver transplantation [6].

No standards exist for hemodynamic monitoring during liver transplantation, but there are a series of options, each with their advantages and disadvantages [7]. The choice depends on the center where the surgical intervention takes place, team experience, economic status, preoperative evaluation and optimization of the patient. The anesthetic consultant makes a personalized decision for appropriate hemodynamic monitoring during liver transplantation.

Our transplant center routinely uses the PiCCO system for hemodynamic monitoring during liver transplantation. It allows cardiac output determination that combines pulse contour analysis and the transpulmonary thermodilution technique. A femoral arterial thermodilution catheter needs to be inserted. One of the advantages is the continuous CO monitoring with pulse contour analysis [8]. Compared to a Swan Ganz pulmonary catheter, the PiCCO system is a less invasive method.

The hemodynamic status of the patient varies between the three important stages of the liver transplant surgery (preanhepatic, anhepatic and neohepatic) and the surgical technique. Preanhepatic stage is the initial stage of liver transplantation where liver dissection takes place. It is associated with a higher risk of bleeding when the patient presents with a history of surgical interventions, previous spontaneous peritonitis, redo liver transplant, portal hypertension or hypervolemia [9].

The anhepatic phase is characterized by the clamping of the portal vein, hepatic artery and suprahepatic veins. It ends with the reperfusion of the graft via the portal vein, in the majority of cases, or hepatic artery. Depending on the surgical technique used, the anhepatic phase can lead to cardiovascular instability due to the blockage of hepatic outflow or inferior vena cava clamping. Severe cardiovascular collapse can be managed with the use of vasoactive drugs, temporary portosystemic shunt or veno-venous bypass [10].

In the neohepatic phase, the graft is being perfused and the new liver slowly restarts its function. During this phase, the postreperfusion syndrome can occur and is characterized with a 30% decrease in arterial pressure for at least a minute during the first 5 min after graft reperfusion [11].

2. Materials and Methods

In this paper, we sought to elucidate some aspects related to the hemodynamic profile of patients with liver cirrhosis and its modification during the three important surgical stages. The objectives of the present study included the characterization of hemodynamic disturbances encountered during liver transplantation with the help of the PiCCO system and their variations during the three surgical stages, the impact of bleeding on hemodynamic status and correlation between the amount of bleeding, lactate levels and survival rate and complications. Another objective was the amount of transfused blood products and their impact on postoperative complications.

In order to achieve the research objectives, the present study included 70 consecutive patients who underwent liver transplantation in the liver transplant center of the Fundeni

Clinical Institute between January and December 2022 and who were hemodynamically monitored invasively through the PiCCO (Pulse Contour Cardiac Output) system. The PiCCO system represents a standard monitoring system for adult liver transplantation in our hospital. Patients under 18 years of age or with incomplete data were excluded. The study was conducted in accordance with the declaration of Helsinki and approved by the Local Ethics Committee (no 16021/23.05.2023).

The inclusion of patients in this study was performed retrospectively and demographic data, laboratory data, severity scores, liver disease etiology, transfusion of blood products as well as hemodynamic parameters measured using the PiCCO device in the three surgical stages (CI, SVRI, GEF; GEDI) were recorded. Hospital protocol involves PiCCO calibration via the transpulmonary thermodilution technique with 20 mL cold saline during each of the three stages of liver transplantation and also every time new hemodynamic changes or instability occur. Recorded PiCCO parameters are averages of calibrated determinations in each of the three stages of liver transplantation.

Postoperative data were also recorded, including the duration of postoperative mechanical ventilation, complications, intensive care unit length of stay and 30/90-day mortality.

For this group of patients studied, different variables that characterize the patients' evolution during different surgical stages were analyzed. A series of variables were collected, including continuous variables (age, Meld severity score, creatinine, duration of surgery, bleeding, etc.), binary variables (sex; 30/90-day survival,) and categorical variables (diagnosis). In order to analyze the connections between these groups of variables, adequate statistical tests were performed. For binary variables, we used the statistical method entitled logistic regression through which we analyzed the way the explicative variable influences the probability of event occurrence expressed as the target variable. For example, the target variable may be the 30-day mortality and the explicative variable may be the Meld score. The logistic regression will estimate the impact of Meld score on the probability of 30-day mortality. Secondary to this estimation, a statistical model arises that explains the relationship between the Meld score and mortality. As a result of the transformations made, with the estimated coefficient and a Meld value, we can estimate the probability of mortality. The quality of this model depends on the Meld value implication in mortality, the number of patients and the sample quality.

When the target variable is continuous, linear regression is used. In this case, the resulting coefficient secondary to logistic regression shows the marginal contribution of the explicative variable on the changes in the target variable. For example, for a coefficient of 5, for the explicative variable, if this increases by 1 unit, the target variable will increase by 5 units.

Every estimated coefficient is tested in order to see to which degree it will be significantly different from 0, meaning if the explicative variable has a real impact on the target value. For this case, we use the t test for linear regression and the z test for logistic regression. Data modeling was performed using the Phyton 3.9 programming language along with the classic modeling packages such as statmodels and the seaborn processing package.

3. Results

Our study included 70 patients, 38 men (54.2%) and 32 women (45.8%) diagnosed with liver cirrhosis and undergoing liver transplant surgery. The median age of the patients is 53.5 years. In total, 27% (19) of the transplanted patients were diagnosed with liver cirrhosis-HCV, 21.5% (15 patients) with liver cirrhosis HBV + HDV, 21.5% (15 patients) with toxic nutritional liver cirrhosis, 7 patients presented Wilson's disease, and 2 patients underwent liver transplantation for acute liver failure.

The mean Meld severity score for liver transplant patients was 18 points. The distribution of the Meld severity score is shown in Figure 1. In the present study, 10 patients were transplanted with a related donor liver segment, and the remaining 60 patients received a brain-dead donor whole liver. The median value of ascites fluid drained intraoperatively was 900 mL. In total, 50% of patients had less than 1000 mL of ascites fluid. The mean duration of surgery was 376 min. A proportion of 44.28% of patients (n = 31) developed complications in the postoperative period.

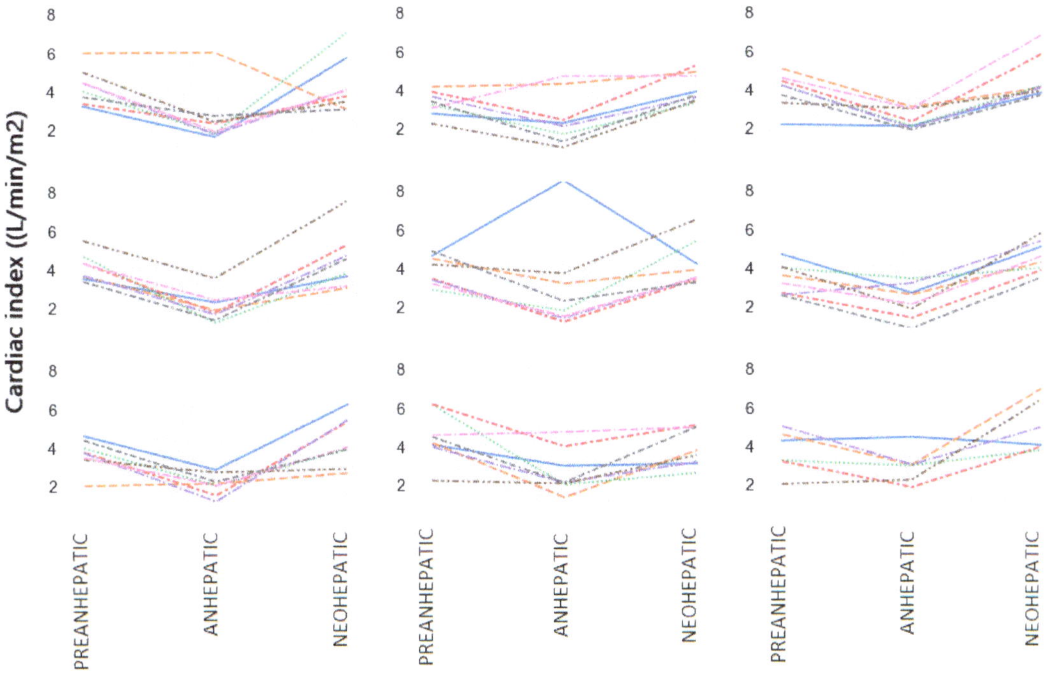

Figure 1. Cardiac index variation. Each line represents a different patient in the figure.

Twelve (35%) patients developed pulmonary complications. Four patients developed pulmonary infection confirmed with signs/symptoms and chest imaging (CT scan or chest radiography) combined with inflammatory markers (C reactive protein, procalcitonin and presepsin), as well as positive cultures. Three patients had acute pulmonary noncardiogenic edema through the transfusion-related acute lung injury mechanism, which happened during blood product transfusion. Two patients developed pulmonary embolism confirmed with a CT scan. Three patients had significant pleural effusion on chest imaging, which needed chest drainage. Five patients developed surgical complications confirmed with a CT scan: Two patients had hemoperitoneum that needed surgical reintervention and three patients suffered complications with abdominal collections that needed CT-guided percutaneous drainage in the interventional radiology laboratory. Four (12%) patients had renal complications, leading to acute kidney injury stage III, which needed continuous veno-venous hemodiafiltration procedures. Three patients had cardiovascular complications: one presented with paroxistic atrial fibrillation on the electrocardiogram and two patients had non-ST elevation myocardial infarction confirmed with transthoracic echocardiography and dynamic changes in cardiac enzymes (hsTnI, CK and CK-MB). Seven patients developed hepatic complications and two patients had primary graft nonfunction (PNF) and liver function inconsistent with life that appeared in the first 7 days. According to strict UNOS criteria, PNF is defined as serum AST levels $\geq$ 3000 U/L associated with at least one of the following: INR $\geq$ 2.5, acidosis corresponding to arterial pH $\leq$ 7.30 or venous pH $\leq$ 7.25 and/or serum lactate levels $\geq$ 4 mmol/L [12]. Other clinical manifestations include persistent encephalopathy and metabolic acidosis, marked hypoglycemia, coagulopathy and reduced or absent bile production associated with a progressive increase in serum AST levels. Once the diagnosis was confirmed and other causes excluded, the patients were subjected to a redo liver transplantation. Two patients developed initial poor graft function, a less severe form of PNF. According to Olthoff et al. [13], using the Pittsburgh definition, initial poor graft function can be diagnosed by meeting at least one of the following criteria: bilirubin concentration ≥ 10 mg/dL on day 7, INR value ≥ 1.6 on day 7, and AST or ALT activity > 2000 U/L in the first 7 days after transplantation. Two patients suffered complications with hepatic artery thrombosis and one patient had right portal vein thrombosis. Three patients developed neurologic complications, including hepatic encephalopathy, which appeared in patients with graft dysfunction. Characteristics of patients who developed postoperative complications and of those who did not develop complications are presented in Table 1.

Table 1. Characteristics of patients with and without postoperative complications.

Variables	Postoperative Complications	
	YES	NO
Bleeding (mL)	9767 (10,099)	2900 (2726)
RBC (units)	9.5 (8.0)	3.1 (3.3)
FFP (units)	12.4 (12)	3.2 (4.4)
Platelets (units)	2. (2.8)	0.7 (1.9)
Cryoprecipitate (units)	1.9 (2.8)	0.6 (1.5)
Fibrinogen (g)	1.6 (2)	0.4 (0.8)
Cold ischemia time (min)	279 (142)	310 (102)
Warm ischemia time (min)	50 (28)	50 (20)
Total transplant time (min)	398 (90)	360 (85)
Reperfusion sindrom	23 patients	21 patients
Anhepatic lactate (mmol)	5.1 (1.9)	3.5 (1.3)
Preanhepatic lactate (mmol)	2.8 (1.3)	2.2 (0.9)
Neohepatic lactate (mmol)	4.7 (2.8)	3.4 (1.5)
CI preanhepatic (L/min/m^2)	4.04 (0.96)	3.75 (0.86)
SVRI preanhepatic (dyne/s/cm^{-5})	1371 (485)	1488 (487)
GEF preanhepatic (%)	35.7 (8.9)	32.2 (5.4)
GEDI preanhepatic (mL/m^2)	697 (181)	648 (152)
CI anhepatic (L/min/m^2)	2.52 (1.09)	2.43 (1.31)
SVRI anhepatic (dyne/s/cm^{-5})	2165 (925)	2909 (1431)
GEF anhepatic (%)	25.6 (6.4)	24.2 (8.3)
GEDI anhepatic (mL/m^2)	653 (178)	553 (131)
CI neohepatic (L/min/m^2)	4.46 (1.2)	4.25 (1.08)
SVRI neohepatic (dyne/s/cm^{-5})	1335 (413)	1431 (336)
GEF neohepatic (%)	33 (6.1)	35.6 (6.6)
GEDI neohepatic (mL/m^2)	720 (203)	673 (139)
Hemoglobin (g/dl)	8.2 (1.3)	8.1 (1.3)
Platelets (/mm^3)	77,354 (59,452)	87,795 (98,606)
INR	2.13 (1.07)	1.9 (0.55)

Values represent mean (SD).

3.1. Variation in the Hemodynamic Parameters during the ThreeImportant Surgical Stages

The surgical technique used in our center consists of inferior vena cava clamping, including supra and infra hepatic clamping, in order to exclude the liver from circulation, which leads to significant venous stasis and compromising heart preload. During the surgical intervention, significant variations in the hemodynamic parameters were observed with a significant decrease in the cardiac index, the global ejection fraction and the global end diastolic volume in the anhepatic stage compared to the pre-anhepatic one.

- Cardiac Index (CI) Variation

The average value of CI in patients in this group in the pre-hepatic phase was 3.88 L/min/m^2, 2.48 L/min/m^2 in the anhepatic stage and 4.36 L/min/m^2 in the neohepatic stage.

A decrease in the CI of approximately 38% is observed in the anhepatic stage as opposed to the pre-anhepaticstage. Also, in the neohepatic stage, there is an increase in the CI by approximately 11% compared to the pre-hepatic stage. The statistical analysis of the parameters measured using the PiCCO system showed that a value within normal limits of the CI (3–4 L/min/m^2) in the pre-hepatic phase was present in 26 patients (37%), and an increased value of over 4 L/ min/m^2 was present in 31 cases (44%). Figure 1 shows the variation in the CI along the three important surgical stages in the 70 patients undergoing liver transplantation.

In the anhepatic phase, all patients showed a significant decrease in cardiac output. In this stage, compared to the pre-hepatic stage, 50% of patients had a decrease of up to 40% in the CI, and the remaining 50% showed decreases of more than 40%. The median value is −0.4, which represents a decrease of 40%. In the neohepatic stage compared to the pre-hepatic stage, 50% of patients had CI increases of more than 10%. In total, 25% of them showed a decrease in the CI, while the remaining 25% had increases of more than 30% (Figure 2).

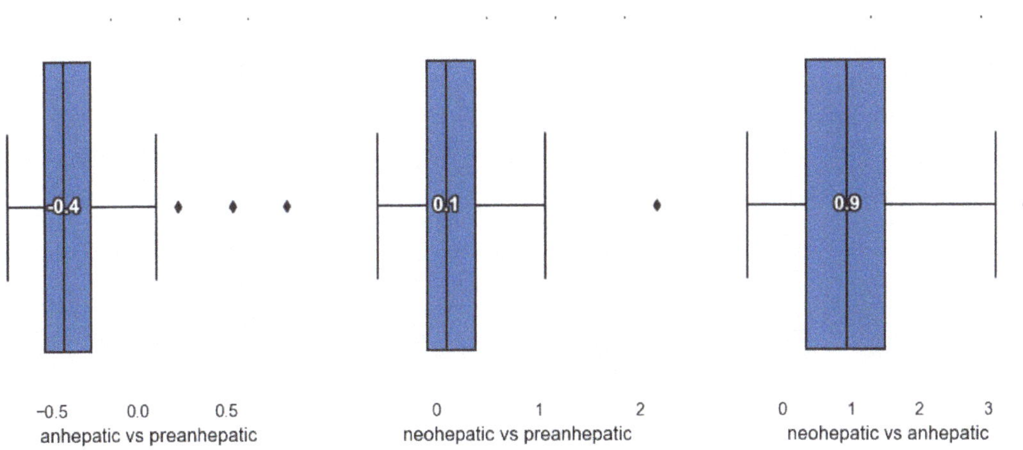

Figure 2. Distribution of cardiac index variation.

In the neohepatic phase compared to the anhepatic stage, it was observed that 50% of the studied patients showed an increase of up to 90% in the CI, and half showed an increase of more than 90% after declamping and reperfusion of the graft.

- Systemic Vascular Resistance Index (SVRI)

The mean value of SVRI was 1439 dynes/s/cm^5/m^2 in the pre-anhepatic stage, 2526 dynes/s/cm^5/m^2 in the anhepatic stage and 1083 dynes/s/cm^5/m^2 in the neohepatic stage. In the neohepatic stage, it was observed that SVRI does not return to the initial value but remains lower. Statistical analysis of the parameters showed that a low value of SVRI (below 1700 dynes/s/cm^5/m^2) in the pre-hepatic phase was present in 40 patients. Figure 3 shows the SVRI variation over the three important surgical stages in the 70 patients undergoing liver transplantation.

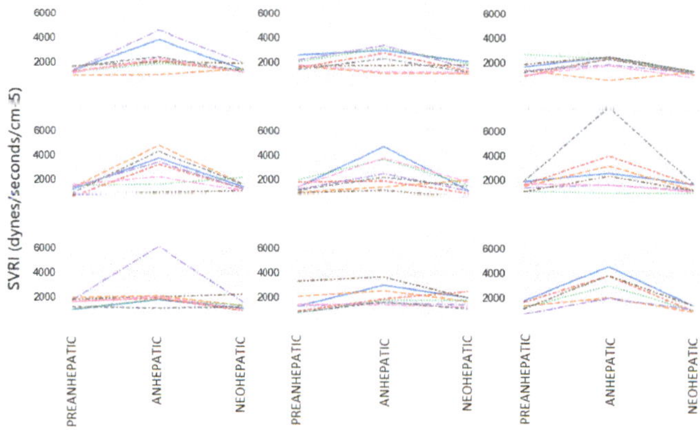

Figure 3. SVRI variation. Each color represents a different patient.

In the anhepatic stage compared to the pre-anhepatic stage, more than 75% of patients show an increase in the SVRI. In total, 50% of patients show increases of more than 60% in the SVRI, while 30% of them show an increase of less than 60%. Less than 25% of the patients show a decrease in the SVRI in the anhepatic stage compared to the pre-anhepatic stage. In the last stage of liver transplantation, the neohepatic compared to the initial, pre-hepatic stage, no significant variation in the SVRI was observed, with 60% of patients registering decreases in the SVRI. In the neohepatic stage, 50% of patients show a decrease of up to 50% in the SVRI compared to the anhepatic stage, and the other half show a decrease of less than 50% (Figure 4).

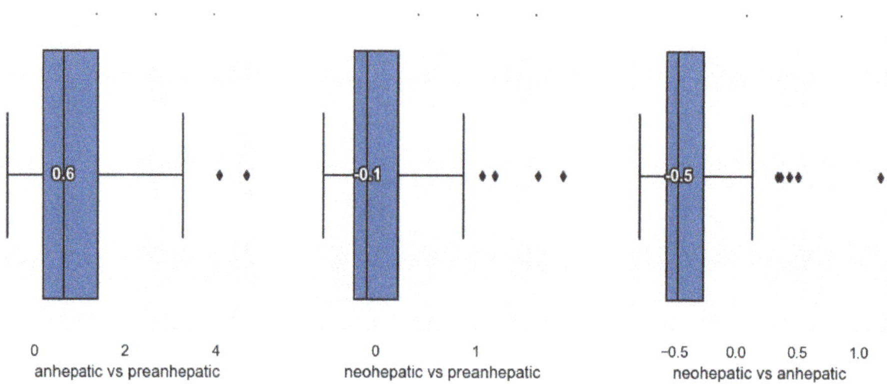

Figure 4. Distribution of SVRI variation.

- Global Ejection Fraction Variation

The average value of GEF in patients from the studied group was 33.7% in the pre-hepatic stage, 25% in the anhepatic stage and 34.5% in the neohepatic stage. The statistical analysis of the determined parameters showed that a normal GEF value (25–35%) in the pre-hepatic phase was present in 65 patients (92.8%), and a low value below 25% was present in 5 cases (7.2%).

In the anhepatic phase compared to the pre-anhepatic one, half of the patients have a decrease in the GEF of more than 30%, and the other half have a decrease of less than 30%. In total, 78% of patients show decreases in global ejection fraction, with a median value of 30%. In the neohepatic stage compared to the initial stage of the transplant, the pre-hepatic stage, 60% of the patients show an increase in the global ejection fraction, with a median value of 10%. In the last stage of the transplant, the neohepatic stage, 85% of the patients show an increase of GEF compared to the anhepatic stage, with a median value of 40% (Figure 5).

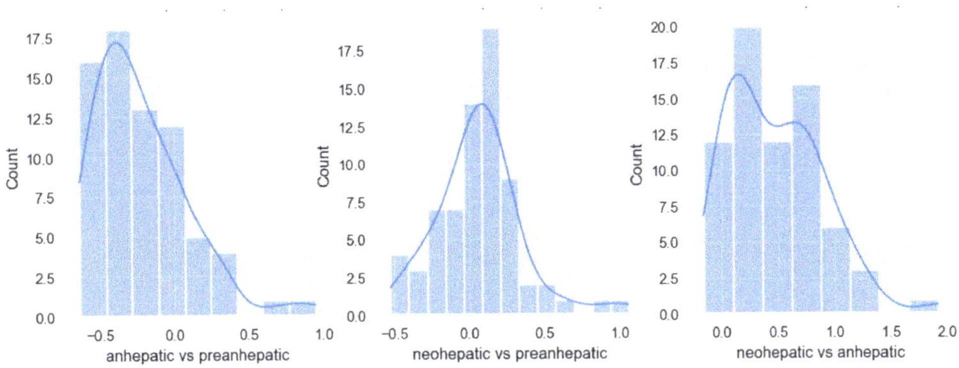

Figure 5. Distribution of GEF variation.

- Noradrenaline Dose Variation

The average value of the noradrenaline dose in the patients in the studied group was 0.22 mcg/kgc/min in the pre-anhepatic stage, 1.04 mcg/kgc/min in the anhepatic stage and 0.22 mcg/kgc/min in the neohepatic stage. Figure 6 shows the variation in noradrenaline dose along the three important surgical stages in the 70 patients undergoing liver transplantation.

In the anhepatic stage compared to the pre-anhepatic stage, all patients register increases in the need for vasopressor support with a median value of 380%. In the neohepatic stage compared to the pre-hepatic one, the dose of noradrenaline is similar to the initial one and the median value of the variation is 0, with approximately 25% of patients registering increases of 150–250% compared to the pre-hepatic stage. In the neohepatic versus the anhepatic stage, all patients experience decreases in noradrenaline dose with a median of 80% (Figure 6).

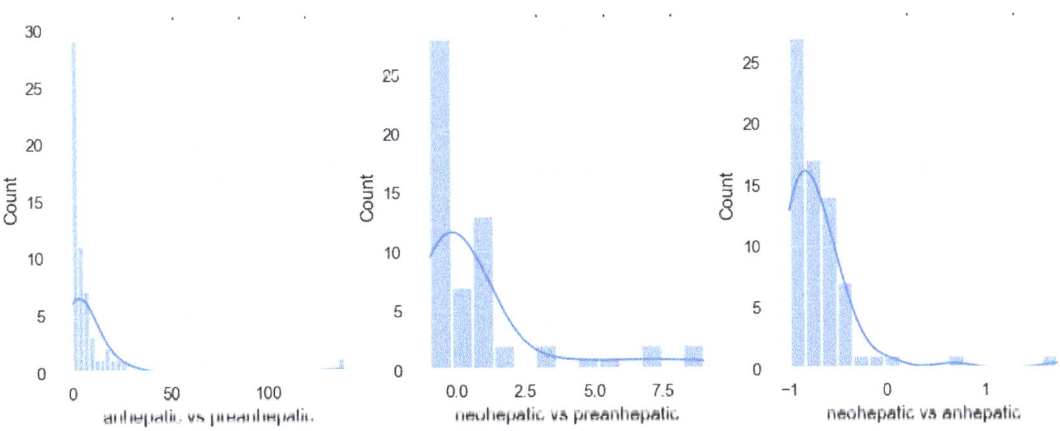

Figure 6. Distribution of noradrenaline variation.

- Variation in Serum Lactate

The average value of serum lactate in the pre-anhepatic stage is 2.49 mmol/L, in the anhepatic stage, it is 4.17 mmol/L, and in the neohepatic stage, the average value is 3.92 mmol/L. Figure 7 shows the variation in serum lactate along the three important surgical stages.

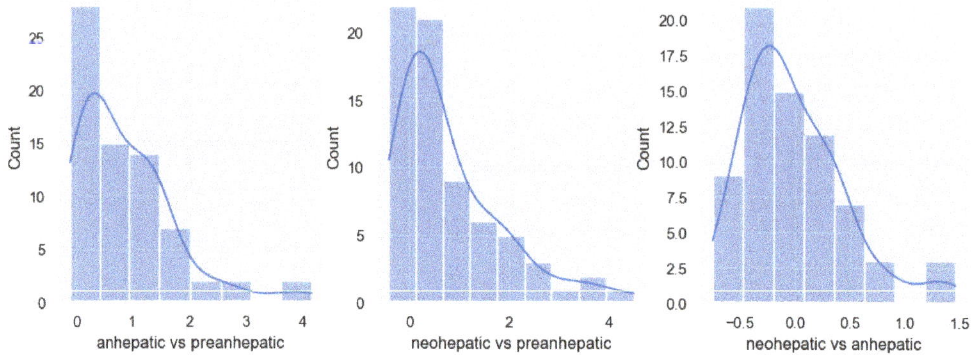

Figure 7. Distribution of lactate variation.

In the anhepatic stage of the transplant, we observe that half of the patients show increases of over 70% in the serum lactate value compared to the initial stage. In total, 98% of all patients show increases in serum lactate at this stage. In the last stage of the surgical intervention, 75% of patients show increases in the value of serum lactate compared to the pre-hepatic stage, with a median value of 40%. The last phase of liver transplantation is characterized by a discrete decrease in the lactate value compared to the anhepatic stage (median value of −10%) (Figure 7).

3.2. Impact of Bleeding on Hemodynamic Status and Postoperative Course

Median intraoperative bleeding is 3000 mL. In total, 75% of the patients in this study have a bleeding amount of less than 6000 mL. Following this graph (Figure 8), it appears that liver transplant patients have a 50% chance of losing an amount of blood below 3000 mL intraoperatively.

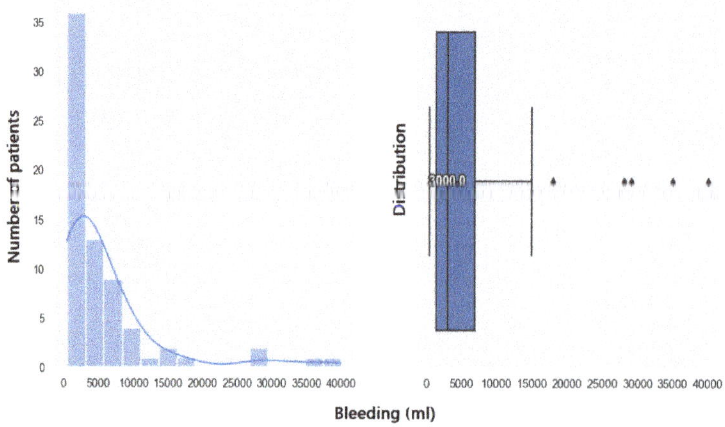

Figure 8. Bleeding distribution.

From the group of patients studied, 31 of them (44.28%) developed immediate postoperative complications. From the distribution pattern below (Figure 9), it can be seen that patients who experienced postoperative complications had a higher degree of intraoperative bleeding.

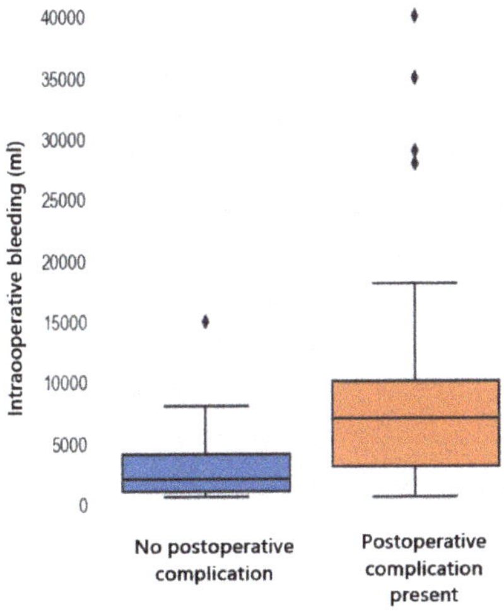

Figure 9. Complications related to bleeding.

To observe the connection between these two variables, i.e., how the bleeding variable affects the postoperative complications variable, we use a logistic regression model. It can be seen that the complications variable is significantly different from 0 because the p-value is 0.002 (below 0.05). Thus, the probability of postoperative complications depending on the amount of bleeding is shown in the graph below.

From the graph below (Figure 10), it can be observed that there is a 50% probability of postoperative complications if the bleeding exceeds 6500mL. In case of a larger amount of bleeding, i.e., 22,000 mL, patients will have an 80% chance of complications after liver transplantation.

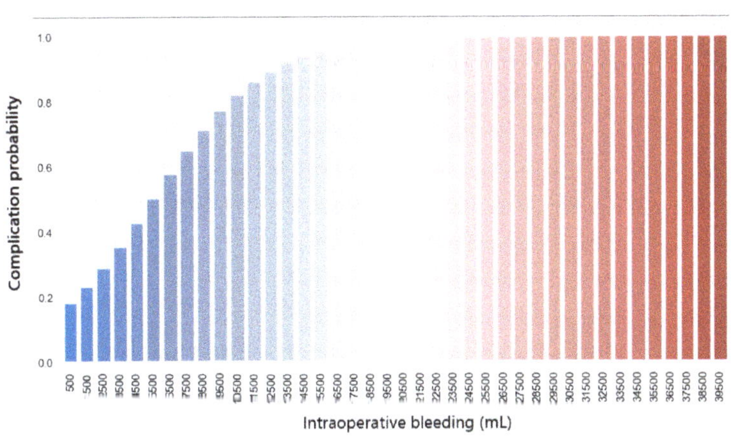

Figure 10. Prediction of complications with regards to bleeding.

In this study group, seven patients (10%) did not survive 30 days after liver transplant surgery. The analysis shows that patients who survive 30 days post-operation have a lower amount of bleeding (Figure 11).

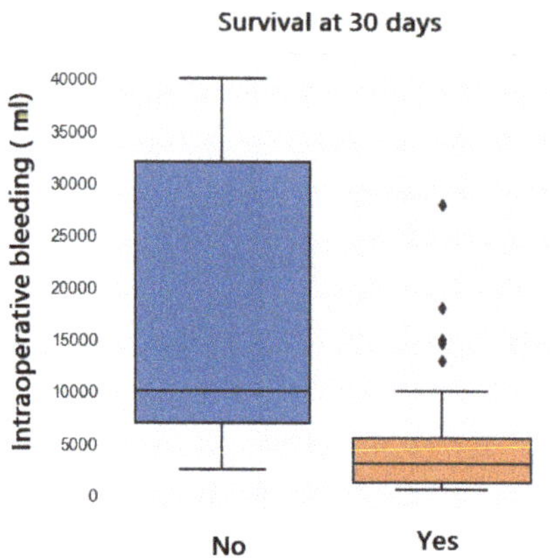

Figure 11. 30-day survival related to bleeding.

To observe the connection between these two variables, i.e., how the bleeding variable affects the 30-day postoperative survival variable, we use a logistic regression model. We observe that the 30-day survival variable is significantly different from 0 because the *p*-value is 0.002 (under 0.05). Thus, the probability of survival at 30 days post-operation according to the amount of bleeding is shown in Figure 12. With a bleed of 10,000 mL, there is a 90% chance of survival at 30 days. In case of a larger amount of bleeding, i.e., 22,000 mL, the chances of survival at 30 days are reduced to 50%.

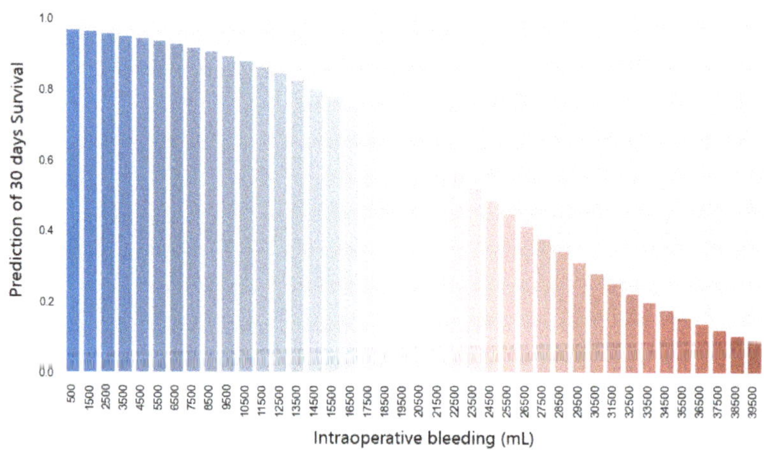

Figure 12. Prediction of 30-daysurvival with regards to bleeding.

In this study group, eight patients (11.42%) did not survive 90 days after liver transplant surgery. Most of the deaths, seven patients (10%), occurred within the first month; thus, this is the critical period after liver transplantation.

To analyze the relationship between these two variables, i.e., how the bleeding variable affects the 90-day postoperative survival variable, we perform a logistic regression model. We observe that the variable survival at 90 days is significantly different from 0 because the p-value is 0.003. With a blood loss of about 5500 mL, there is a 92% chance of survival at 90 days. In case of a larger amount of bleeding, i.e., 10,000 mL, the chances of survival are reduced to 82%. A major bleed of about 20,000 mL will decrease the chances of 90-day survival by 50% (Figure 13).

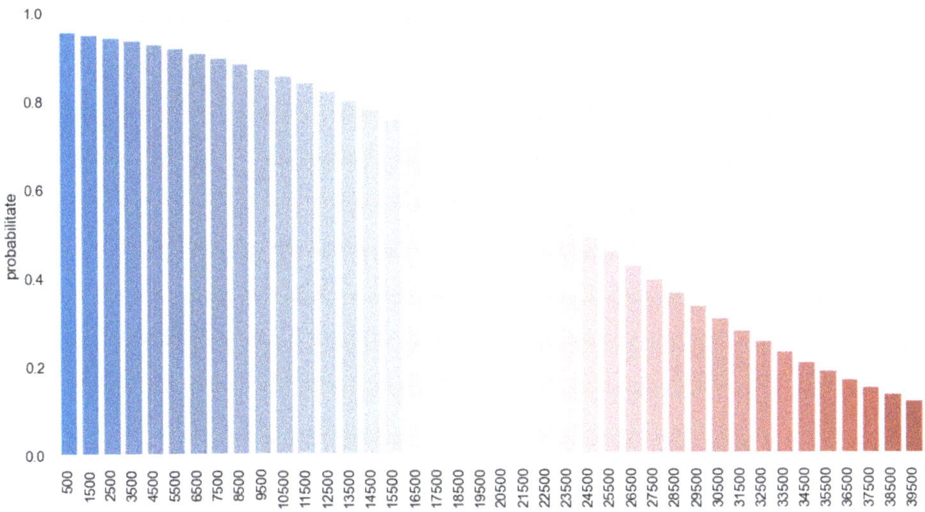

Figure 13. Prediction of 90-daysurvival with regards to bleeding.

Logistic regression was performed to confirm if intraoperative bleeding relates to the length of intensive care unit stay. It can be seen that the length of ICU stay is not influenced by the amount of intraoperative bleeding; it is not a statistically significant relationship (p-value 0.239).

Patients in the study group had a median Meld score of 19 points. A correlation between Meld score and intraoperative bleeding was observed. The logistic regression confirms the statistical importance ($p = 0.01$). Bleeding variation is explained by 9% of the preoperative severity score.

3.3. The Impact of Serum Lactate on Outcome of Transplanted Patients

The median value of anhepatic serum lactate is 3.8 mmol/L. In total, 50% of patients have serum lactate values above 5 mmol/L in the anhepatic phase. Figure 14 shows the correlation between anhepatic lactate and intraoperative bleeding.

The logistic regression model shows that intraoperative bleeding is responsible for 13% of the variation in the anhepatic lactate level ($p = 0.002$).

The median length of intensive care unit (ICU) stay is 6 days. Anhepatic lactate correlates with the ICU length of stay. It increases by 0.53 each time the lactate increases by 1 unit. The logistic regression shows that the ICU length of stay is explained with a proportion of 9% by the anhepatic lactate variable ($p = 0.012$).

The present study also looked at neohepatic lactate and its impact on outcome. Neohepatic lactate does not correlate with the prolonged ICU length of stay ($p = 0.17$). Patients who developed postoperative complications had higher levels of neohepatic lactate compared to those without complications. The regression tests showed how neohepatic lactate affects the rate of postoperative complications ($p = 0.033$). The probability of complications depending on the value of neohepatic lactate is shown in Figure 15. A lactate level of 5 mmol/L is associated with a 50% chance of postoperative complications.

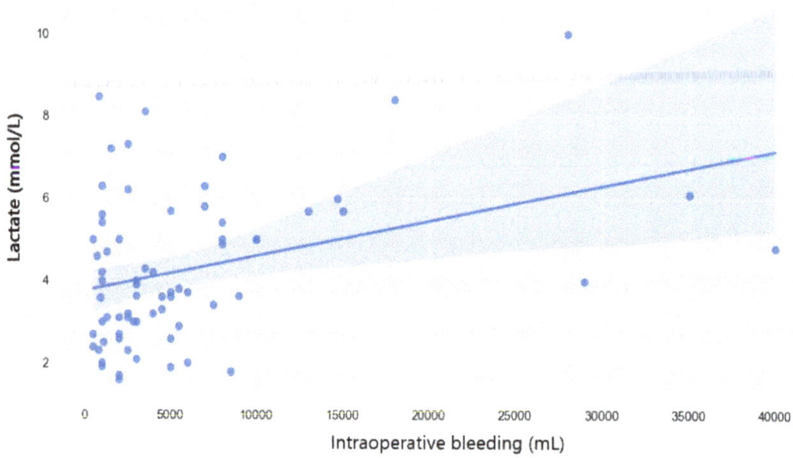

Figure 14. Correlation between anhepatic lactate and intraoperative bleeding.

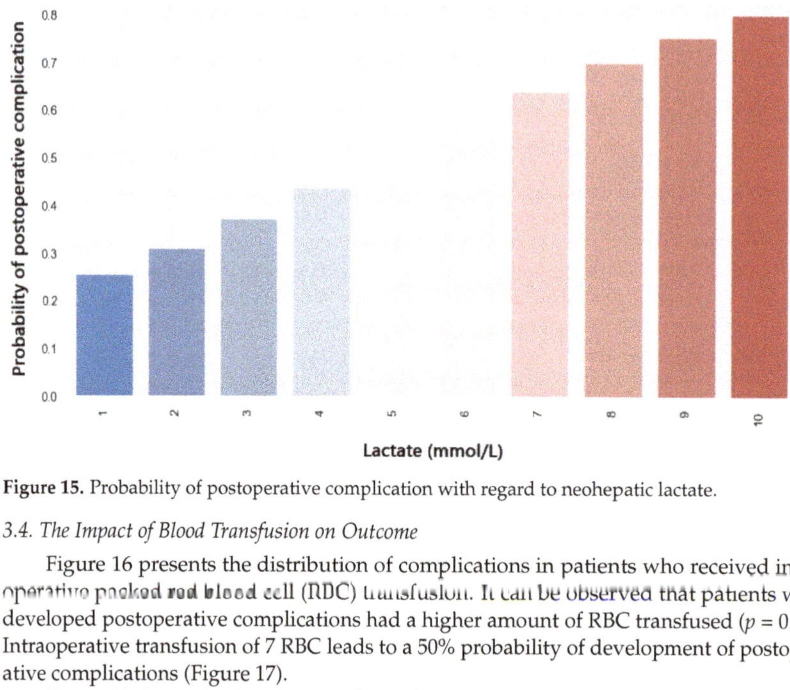

Figure 15. Probability of postoperative complication with regard to neohepatic lactate.

3.4. The Impact of Blood Transfusion on Outcome

Figure 16 presents the distribution of complications in patients who received intraoperative packed red blood cell (RBC) transfusion. It can be observed that patients who developed postoperative complications had a higher amount of RBC transfused ($p = 0.05$). Intraoperative transfusion of 7 RBC leads to a 50% probability of development of postoperative complications (Figure 17).

Figure 18 shows the distribution of complications in patients who received intraoperative fresh frozen plasma (FFP). Patients who developed complications had a higher amount of FFP transfused ($p = 0.001$). The transfusion of 5 units of FFP will lead to a 40% chance of development of postoperative complications (Figure 19).

The same tests were performed for cryoprecipitate and platelets. Statistical analysis showed that there is no correlation between these blood products and the appearance of postoperative complications.

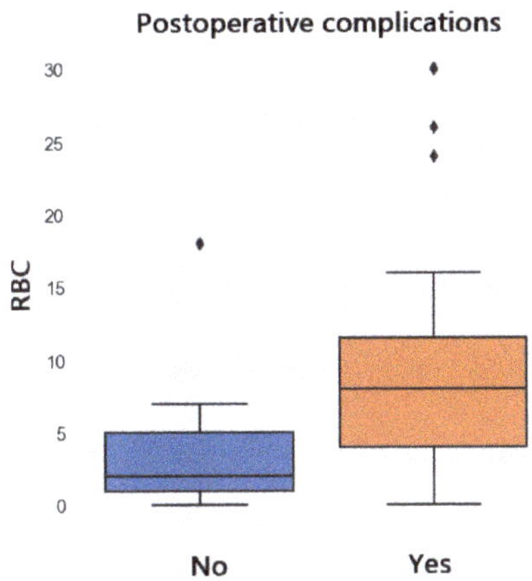

Figure 16. Complications related to RBC transfusion.

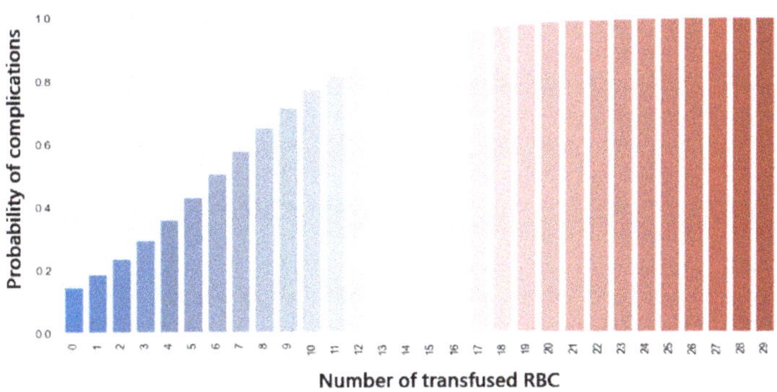

Figure 17. Probability of complications with regard to PRBC.

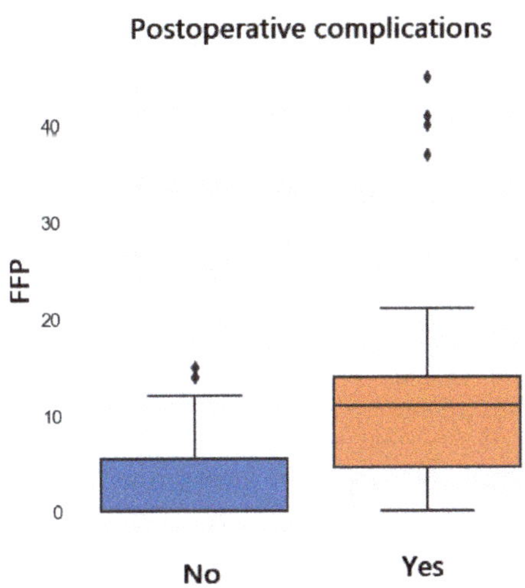

Figure 18. Postoperative complications and FFP transfusion.

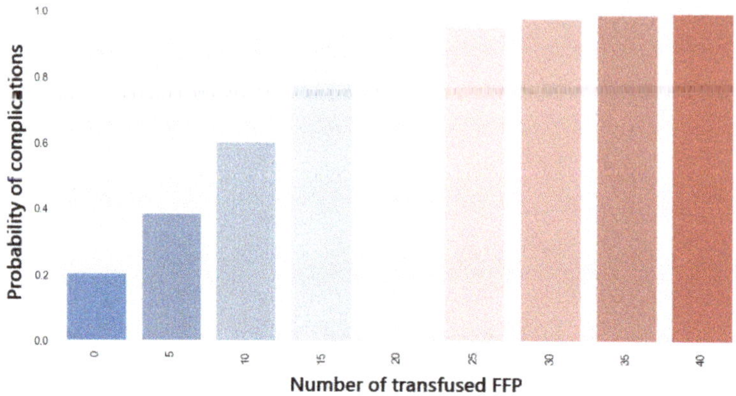

Figure 19. Probability of complications related to FFP transfusion.

4. Discussion

Liver transplantation is the treatment of choice for end-stage liver disease. The Meld score is used all over the world for liver graft allocation. The present thesis reports the variation in hemodynamic parameters determined with the help of the PiCCO system during the three important surgical stages of liver transplantation.

The literature presents various surgical techniques that can be used during liver transplantation [14]. The surgical technique routinely used in our center involves total IVC clamping with an important decrease in preload and cardiac output with implications for cardiovascular status and anesthetic management. The invasive cardiac output monitoring system is extremely important during liver transplantation due to the marked hemodynamic instability that can occur and can provide us with additional information related to cardiac output, dosing of vasopressor/inotropic substances and as guiding volume management and patients' response to volume repletion. The study showed that in the anhepatic phase, there is an important decrease in the cardiac output, the global ejection fraction and the global end-diastolic volume. Half of the patients present a decrease in the CI with more than 40%. In the neohepatic stage, more than half of the studied patients present a value of cardiac output 10% higher compared to the value in the pre-hepatic phase due to the comeback of the venous return.

As a result of significant variations in CO, there are variations in SVRI. In total, 40 patients present a typical cirrhotic hiperdynamic status, with high CO and low SVRI values [15]. The anhepatic phase results in an important SVRI increase. The present literature advises using the piggyback technique for liver transplantation for better hemodynamic stability. It also suggests the use of veno-venous bypass in case of significant bleeding, hemodynamic instability or severe portal hypertension. One of the particularities of this study is the fact that our center does not use the piggyback technique; thus, hemodynamic instability must be accordingly managed by the consultant anesthetist.

Noradrenaline is the preferred vasopressor used and its variation is consistent with the hemodynamic status during the three surgical stages, including the anhepatic stage that requires high doses to maintain the mean arterial pressure and cardiac output [16].

Intraoperative blood loss can be secondary to impaired liver synthesis, portal hypertension, portal vein thrombosis or splenomegaly. All these factors associated with surgical technique can lead to significant blood loss and blood transfusion [17]. Despite recent progress, liver transplantation remains a surgical act with a high risk of bleeding [17].

Similar to the literature data, our study showed that intraoperative bleeding influences the outcome of transplant patients and there is a 50% chance of postoperative complications if bleeding exceeds 6500 mL. Most of the deaths occurred within 1 month postoperatively, which is the critical period after liver transplantation. With a blood loss of about 5500 mL, there is a 92% chance of 90-day survival. Intraoperative bleeding requires intraoperative transfusion with products such as PRBC, FFP, cryoprecipitate or platelets. Similar to the literature data, our study showed that RBC and FFP transfusion are associated with postoperative complications and prolonged mechanical ventilation. Due to the well-known side effects blood transfusion might have on patients, our center guides intraoperative transfusion with the use of viscoelastic tests—rotational thromboelastometry.

Statistical tests performed on this group of patients provided information related to the probability of 30/90-day survival and the occurrence of complications according to variables such as intraoperative bleeding and Meld severity score. Also, the anhepatic and neohepatic lactate values provide information related to the probability of complications and graft dysfunction. Increased intraoperative lactate values are a marker of tissue anoxia and liver graft dysfunction. Hyperlactatemia at the end of surgery has been demonstrated to correlate with an increase in 30- and 90-day mortality [18].

Studies show that the majority of complications occur during the first 3 months after liver transplantation [19].

The results of the present study open new hypotheses for future studies regarding hemodynamic monitoring of cardiac output during liver transplantation. The usefulness of transesophageal ultrasound in comparison with invasive means of monitoring of the hemodynamic status will be the focus of our next study.

5. Conclusions

The present paper investigates the hemodynamic status of liver transplant patients and their variation during the three stages of surgical intervention. The PiCCO system proved a useful tool for CO measurement and management during liver transplant. Considering the IVC clamping and the total blood loss, important hemodynamic variations were present during the three surgical phases, with the anhepatic stage being the most unstable with high noradrenaline doses. All patients presented a decrease in cardiac output and global ejection fraction in the anhepatic phase. Accurate hemodynamic management is necessary during this high-risk procedure on cirrhotic patients. Intraoperative bleeding has a major impact on patients' outcomes and the first month represents a critical period after liver transplantation. Intraoperative transfusion correlates with the occurrence of postoperative complications.

The present study has its limitations. It is a retrospective study and the total number of patients included is quite small. The lack of another cardiac monitoring device is another limitation of the study.

Author Contributions: Conceptualization: L.N.B.; Methodology: L.N.B., C.L.A. and C.E.J.; Software: O.C.; Validation: C.L.A.; Formal analysis: L.N.B., C.E.J. and O.C.; Investigation: L.N.B. and C.E.J.; Writing—original draft preparation: L.N.B. and C.D.; Writing—review and editing: O.C.; Visualization: C.L.A.; Supervision: G.D. All authors have read and agreed to the published version of the manuscript.

Funding: This research received no external funding.

Institutional Review Board Statement: The study was conducted according to the guidelines of the Declaration of Helsinki. Our research in the hospital and data extraction from the hospital archive were approved by the Medical and Health Service Manager of the Fundeni Clinical Institute.This is a non-interventional study that only entails data collection andethical approval was grantedby Ethics Committee of Fundeni Clinical Institute (no 16021/23.05.2023).

Informed Consent Statement: Patient consent was waived due to the fully anonymized and observational design of the study.

Data Availability Statement: The data presented in this study are available upon request from the corresponding author. The data are not publicly available due to ethical restrictions.

Conflicts of Interest: The authors declare no conflicts of interest.

References

1. Kalluru, R.; Gadde, S.; Chikatimalla, R.; Dasaradhan, T.; Koneti, J.; Cherukuri, S.P. Cirrhotic Cardiomyopathy: The Interplay Between Liver and Heart. *Cureus* **2022**, *14*, e27969. [CrossRef]
2. Tovikkai, C.; Charman, S.C.; Praseedom, R.K.; Gimson, A.E.; van der Meulen, J. Time-varying impact of comorbidities on mortality after liver transplantation: A national cohort study using linked clinical and administrative data. *BMJ Open* **2015**, *5*, e006971. [CrossRef] [PubMed]
3. Moller, S.; Lee, S.S. Cirrhotic cardiomyopathy. *J. Hepatol.* **2018**, *69*, 958–960. [CrossRef]
4. Chayanupatkul, M.; Liangpunsakul, S. Cirrhotic cardiomyopathy: Review of pathophysiology and treatment. *Hepatol. Int.* **2014**, *8*, 308–315. [CrossRef]
5. Rudnick, M.R.; Marchi, L.D.; Plotkin, J.S. Hemodynamic monitoring during liver transplantation: A state of the art review. *World J. Hepatol.* **2015**, *7*, 1302–1311. [CrossRef]
6. Jung, J.-Y.; Sohn, J.Y.; Lim, L.; Cho, H.; Ju, J.-W.; Yoon, H.-K.; Yang, S.-M.; Lee, H.-J.; Kim, W.H. Pulmonary artery catheter monitoring versus arterial waveform-based monitoring during liver transplantation: A retrospective cohort study. *Sci. Rep.* **2023**, *13*, 19947. [CrossRef]
7. Feltracco, P.; Biancofiore, G.L.; Ori, C.; Saner, F.H.; Della Rocca, G. Limits and pitfalls of haemodynamic monitoring systems in liver transplantation surgery. *Minerva Anesthesiol.* **2012**, *78*, 1372–1384.
8. Lee, M.; Weinberg, L.; Pearce, B.; Scurrah, N.; Story, D.A.; Pillai, P.; McCall, P.R.; McNicol, L.P.; Peyton, P.J. Agreement in hemodynamic monitoring during orthotopic liver transplantation: A comparison of Flo Trac/Vigileo at two monitoring sites with pulmonary artery catheter thermodilution. *J. Clin. Monit. Comput.* **2017**, *31*, 343–351. [CrossRef] [PubMed]
9. Brezeanu, L.N.; Brezeanu, R.C.; Diculescu, M.; Droc, G. Anaesthesia for liver transplantation: An update. *J. Crit. Care Med.* **2020**, *6*, 91–100. [CrossRef] [PubMed]
10. Lapisatepun, W.; Lapisatepun, W.; Agopian, V.; Xia, V.W. Venovenous Bypass During Liver Transplantation: A New Look at an Old Technique. *Transplant. Proc.* **2020**, *52*, 905–909. [CrossRef] [PubMed]
11. Sahmeddini, M.A.; Tehran, S.G.; Khosravi, M.B.; Eghbal, M.H.; Asmarian, N.; Khalili, F.; Vatankhah, P.; Izadi, S. Risk factors of the post-reperfusion syndrome during orthotopic liver transplantation: A clinical observational study. *BMC Anesthesiol.* **2022**, *22*, 89. [CrossRef]
12. Al-Freah, M.A.B.; McPhail, M.J.W.; Dionigi, E.; Foxton, M.R.; Auzinger, G.; Rela, M.; Wendon, J.A.; O'Grady, J.G.; Heneghan, M.A.; Heaton, N.D.; et al. Improving the diagnostic criteria for primary liver graft nonfunction in adults utilizing standard and transportable laboratory parameters: An outcome-based analysis. *Am. J. Transplant.* **2017**, *17*, 1255–1266. [CrossRef] [PubMed]
13. Olthoff, K.M.; Kulik, L.; Samstein, B.; Kaminski, M.; Abecassis, M.; Emond, J.; Shaked, A.; Christie, J.D. Validation of a current definition of early allograft dysfunction in liver transplant recipients and analysis of risk factors. *Liver Transplant.* **2010**, *16*, 943–949. [CrossRef]
14. Chen, Z.; Ju, W.; Chen, C.; Wang, T.; Yu, J.; Hong, X.; Dong, Y.; Chen, M.; He, X. Application of various surgical techniques in liver transplantation: A retrospective study. *Ann. Transl. Med.* **2021**, *9*, 1367. [CrossRef] [PubMed]
15. Villanueva, C.; Albillos, A.; Genesca, J.; Abraldes, J.G.; Calleja, J.L.; Aracil, C.; Bañares, R.; Morillas, R.; Poca, M.; Peñas, B.; et al. Development of hyperdynamic circulation and response to beta-blockers in compensated cirrhosis with portal hypertension. *Hepatology* **2016**, *63*, 197–206. [CrossRef] [PubMed]
16. Taura, P.; Martinez-Palli, G.; Blasi, A.; Rivas, E.; Beltran, J.; Balust, J. Intraoperative Management of High-Risk Liver Transplant Re-cipients: Concerns and Challenges. *Transplant. Proc.* **2016**, *48*, 2491–2494. [CrossRef] [PubMed]
17. Kasraian, L.; Nikeghbalian, S.; Karimi, M.H. Blood product transfusion in liver transplantation and its impact on short-term survival. *Int. J. Org. Transplant Med.* **2018**, *9*, 105–111.
18. Takahashi, K.; Jafri, S.R.; Safwan, M.; Abouljoud, M.S.; Nagai, S. Peri-transplant lactate levels and delayed lactate clearance as predictive factors for poor outcomes after liver transplantation: A propensity score–matched study. *Clin. Transplant.* **2019**, *33*, e13613. [CrossRef] [PubMed]
19. Mueller, A.R.; Platz, K.P.; Kremer, B. Early postoperative complications following liver transplantation. *Best. Pract. Res. Clin. Gastroenterol.* **2004**, *18*, 881–900. [CrossRef] [PubMed]

Journal of *Personalized Medicine*

MDPI

Article

The Effectiveness of Adipose Tissue-Derived Mesenchymal Stem Cells Mixed with Platelet-Rich Plasma in the Healing of Inflammatory Bowel Anastomoses: A Pre-Clinical Study in Rats

Georgios Geropoulos [1], Kyriakos Psarras [1,*], Maria Papaioannou [2], Vasileios Geropoulos [1], Argyri Niti [3], Christina Nikolaidou [4], Georgios Koimtzis [1], Nikolaos Symeonidis [1], Efstathios T. Pavlidis [1], Georgios Koliakos [3], Theodoros E. Pavlidis [1] and Ioannis Galanis [1]

1 2nd Propaedeutical Department of Surgery, Hippokration Hospital, School of Medicine, Aristotle University of Thessaloniki, 54642 Thessaloniki, Greece; drgxkoimtzis@gmail.com (G.K.); niksym@gmail.com (N.S.); pavlidis.md@gmail.com (E.T.P.); pavlidth@auth.gr (T.E.P.); galanis@auth.gr (I.G.)
2 Laboratory of Biological Chemistry, School of Medicine, Aristotle University of Thessaloniki, 54124 Thessaloniki, Greece; mpapaioannou@auth.gr
3 Biohellenika Biotechnology Company, 55535 Thessaloniki, Greece; argyrw.niti@gmail.com (A.N.)
4 Department of Histopathology, Hippokration Hospital, 54642 Thessaloniki, Greece; christinapathologist@gmail.com
* Correspondence: psarrask@auth.gr; Tel.: +30-2310892182

Abstract: Introduction: Multiple factors have been linked with increased risk of anastomotic leak in bowel surgery, including infections, inflammatory bowel disease, patient comorbidities and poor surgical technique. The aim of this study was to investigate the positive effect, if any, of adipose derived mesenchymal stem cells (MSCs) mixed with platelet-rich plasma (PRP) in the healing of bowel anastomoses, in an inflammatory environment after establishment of experimental colitis. **Materials and Methods:** Thirty-five male Wistar rats were divided into five groups of seven animals: normal controls, colitis controls, PRP, MSCs, and PRP+MSCs. All groups underwent laparotomy, one-cm segmental colectomy and anastomosis in situ. In the colitis group, colectomy was performed at the affected area. Colitis was previously established by transrectal administration of 2,4,6-trinitrobenzene sulfonic acid (TNBS) except for the normal controls. Post-mortem histopathological, tissue hydroxyproline and anastomotic bursting pressure (ABP) assessments were performed. The Mann–Whitney U test was used to assess statistical significance differences between groups. **Results:** No perioperative mortality was noted. Tissue hydroxyproline and ABP were significantly increased in the group of PRP+MSCs compared to colitis controls ($p = 0.0151$ and $p = 0.0104$, respectively). Inflammatory cell infiltration was lower and fibroblast activity higher in PRP+MSCs group, but not statistically significant ($p > 0.05$). Neoangiogenesis ($p = 0.0073$) and anastomotic area epithelialization ($p = 0.0182$) were significantly higher in PRP + MSCs group compared to colitis controls. **Discussion:** The synergistic effect of the PRP and MSCs is apparently responsible for the improved healing markers in bowel anastomoses even on inflammatory bowel. This gives hope for primary anastomoses and stoma saving in many emergency and/or elective circumstances, especially in immunocompromised or malnourished patients, even in cases with inflammation or peritonitis. Clinical studies should follow in order to support the clinical application of PRP+MSCs in gastrointestinal anastomoses.

Keywords: mesenchymal stem cells; platelet-rich plasma; anastomosis; intestinal healing; anastomotic leak; colitis

1. Introduction

Despite our extended knowledge of the healing process in the gastrointestinal wall, the anastomotic leak is still a major problem in clinical practice. Even after meticulous patient preparation and optimization of factors like anastomotic technique, patient comorbidities and perioperative care, anastomotic leakage may occur in up to 14% of cases but varies depending on the location of the anastomosis and the participating organs [1–3]. For example, leakage rates may be up to 17.5% in pancreaticojejunal, 14.6% in esophagojejunal and up to 17% in ileocecal anastomoses [4–6]. In cases where the patient presents any reasons for bad healing (elderly, immunocompromised, malnourished, inflammation, infection, etc.), a bowel anastomosis may lead to a detrimental series of septic complications if a leakage occurs. This is riskier in emergency settings with unprepared bowel or in inflammation sites (inflammatory bowel or peritonitis). To avoid such complications, most surgeons prefer to avoid the anastomosis itself by changing the operation to Hartmann's procedure, or, if they decide to complete the anastomosis in the first setting, most of them choose to establish a prophylactic stoma or ileostomy. Stomas may sound a safe option for the surgeon; however they are not free of complications, and many patients find it quite frustrating, with negative impact on their quality of life [7].

Adipose tissue is an excellent source of mesenchymal stem cells (MSCs), given its abundance in humans and experimental animals. Adipose tissue-derived MSCs have been proven to provide a significant benefit in wound healing via several mechanisms. MSCs secrete significant levels of growth factors, extracellular matrix and cytokines that modulate the immune function [8,9]. Following tissue damage stimuli, a variety of growth factors, including tumor necrosis factor-α (TNF-α), fibroblast growth factor (FGF), vascular endothelial growth factor (VEGF) and transforming growth factor-β (TGF-β) are released. These growth factors have been repeatedly shown to significantly enhance wound healing [8,10]. At sites of tissue damage, the recruited MSCs express the C-X-C chemokine receptor type 4 (CXCR-4) protein, which twists inflammatory cells to present an enhanced wound healing activity [11]. The extracellular matrix proteins secreted by MSCs assist in the angiogenesis and chemotaxis of inflammatory cells that promote wound healing. MSCs constitute 1% of the adipose tissue cellular population. Additionally, MSCs participate in the wound healing process by differentiating into fibroblasts and epithelial cells, and they substitute tissue damage by tissue regeneration via a series of multiple actions mediated by certain receptors and pathways. Moreover, the growth factors secreted by MSCs stimulate cells adjacent to tissue injury to participate in the wound healing process [12]. It is very important that MSCs do not provoke immune reactions, since they do not express any histocompatibility complex antigens. Interestingly, previous studies have shown that when MSCs are incorporated into other biomaterials like chitosan, enhance wound healing by their ability to differentiate into epithelial cells [13]. Furthermore, exosomes and microvesicles secreted by MSCs induce cell migration and wound matrix remodeling with an increased production of collagen [14]. These characteristics make MSCs a valuable tool to use in multiple clinical scenarios.

Platelet-rich plasma (PRP) is produced from blood via simple centrifugation. Several reports have shown that PRP supports wound healing via its high concentration in various growth factors and cytokines including platelet-derived growth factor (PDGF), TGF-β, FGF, VEGF, hepatocyte growth factor (HGF), insulin-like growth factor (IGF), interleukin-1β, interleukin-6 and interleukin-4 [15,16]. PDGF has been shown to improve epithelialization and tissue regeneration via secretion of several other tissue growth factors [17]. Other studies investigating the combination of PRP and MSCs (PRP+MSCs) have demonstrated that VEGF facilitates MSCs' angiogenic properties and enhances the wound healing process. Finally, fibroblast mitogenic activity is improved by the presence of IGF, which is secreted by PRP [18].

To date, limited literature exists investigating the effect of MSCs or PRP in gastrointestinal wound healing and especially in bowel anastomoses in colitis settings. A very well-established inflammatory bowel disease model is colitis induced via intrarectal administration of 2,4,6- trinitrobenzene sulfonic acid (TNBS), and a wide variety of studies investigating multiple agents in bowel anastomoses healing have been published since [19]. TNBS facilitates Th1 immunologic response and T cell-mediated immune reaction in the exposed tissues, mimicking inflammatory bowel syndromes. Inflammation impairs intestinal wound healing, and wise surgeons would never dare to perform anastomoses in such cases. Therefore, it would be extremely useful to discover ways to enhance healing in inflammatory bowel tissues. This study aims to investigate the healing effectiveness of the combined administration of PRP and MSCs in anastomoses performed in rats with inflammatory bowel disease.

2. Materials and Methods

2.1. Experimental Animals and Study Groups

The animal study protocol was approved by the Institutional Review Board (protocol code EL-54-BIOexp-10 and date of approval 11 September 2023). Forty male Wistar–albino rats of the same age and body weight were used. The first five rats were the donors for adipose tissue and blood in order to prepare the adipose-derived MSCs and the PRP samples. Rats were maintained separately in cages at 22 °C ± 2 °C and 40–50% humidity with a 12-h light/dark cycle and were allowed free access to tap water and standard laboratory rat pellets. Thirty-five rats were randomly divided into five groups of seven rats each: Group 1: end-to-end colonic anastomosis without experimental colitis, Group 2: experimental colitis + end-to-end colonic anastomosis, Group 3: experimental colitis +end-to-end colonic anastomosis +PRP injection, Group 4: experimental colitis+end-to-end colonic anastomosis +MSCs injection and Group 5: experimental colitis +end-to-end colonic anastomosis + PRP+MSCs injection. The G*Power statistical software (software (Faul, Erdfelder, Lang, & Buchner, 2007, version 3.1.9.6) was used to calculate the sample size.

2.2. PRP Preparation

For the purpose of this study, allogeneic PRP was used. A small amount of peripheral blood, approximately 3 mL, was collected from each one of the donors into sterile tubes with EDTA. The tubes were centrifuged for 15 min at $270\times g$, at room temperature. The supernatant was aspirated, and a second centrifugation was executed at $1000\times g$ for 7 min, at room temperature. The platelet-poor plasma was discarded, and the pellet was resuspended in EDTA. The PRP was then transferred into cryogenic tubes and stored at −80 °C in 500 μL aliquots. The final volume of platelet-rich plasma that was injected to each anastomosis was 500 μL divided at four sites in each intestinal stump. This corresponded to a total platelet number of 1×10^6 cells/μL. The purpose of the cryopreservation was the induction of platelet activation and alpha-granule release. Frozen PRP was thawed prior to anastomosis application.

2.3. Isolation, Characterization, and Culture of Adipose Tissue MSCs

The source of adipose tissue and MSCs was allogeneic. Adipose tissue was removed via lipectomy surgeries from the same five donors as aboved and transferred into sterile containers under aseptic conditions. Approximately 2 g of adipose tissue of each sample was cut into fine pieces, washed with normal saline 0.9% to remove red blood cells and digested with 0.075% collagenase type I (Worthington, Columbus, OH, USA) and 1% (*v*/*v*) penicillin/streptomycin (Pen/Strep, Biowest, Nuaillé, France) for 1 h at 37 °C on a shaker. Then, collagenase was removed via dilution with phosphate-buffered saline solution (PBS). The resulting cell suspension was centrifuged at $600\times g$ for 20 min. The supernatant was removed, and the pellet was resuspended in low-glucose Dulbecco's Modified Eagle's Medium (DMEM, Biowest®) supplemented with 10% (*v*/*v*) fetal bovine serum (FBS, Biowest®) and 1% (*v*/*v*) Pen/Strep. Isolated cells were multiplied in T150 flasks using low-glucose DMEM 10% (*v*/*v*) FBS and 1% (*v*/*v*) Pen/Strep at 37 °C in a humid atmosphere containing 5% CO_2 for 7 days. After that, cells were cultured for 7 more days in T75 flasks and finally were stored in cryovials in vapor-phase liquid nitrogen below −150 °C. Flow cytometry analysis showed MSCs to be positive for the expression markers CD90 and CD105. The percentages of positive cell markers and their histograms are given in Figure 1. Moreover, the isolated cells were found to be capable of differentiating into osteocytes, chondrocytes and adipocytes under the appropriate conditions (Figure 1). Differentiation into chondrocytes is shown with production of deposits of acid mucopolysaccharides which were confirmed via Alcian Blue, differentiation into osteoblasts was demonstrated via detection of Alizarin Red S stain-positive calcium deposits, and differentiation into adipocytes was revealed via the formation of cytoplasmic lipid droplets stained with Oil Red O stain (Figure 2). Finally, the stem cells were placed in one-mL microneedle insulin syringes suspended in 500 μL PBS containing 3×10^6 MSCs before their injection into colonic anastomoses circumferentially located at four sites in each intestinal stump. When PRP+MSCs were applied, MSCs were resuspended directly in 500 μL PRP aliquots. Cell viability was checked before injection into the rats. After thawing, a small amount of the cell suspension was used for flow cytometry to determine viability using FITC Annexin V Apoptosis Detection Kit with 7-AAD (EXBIO, Chemical company, Greece)). Fluorescent intensities of the cells were detected using a flow cytometer BD FACSCalibur (BD Biosciences) (Figure 3).

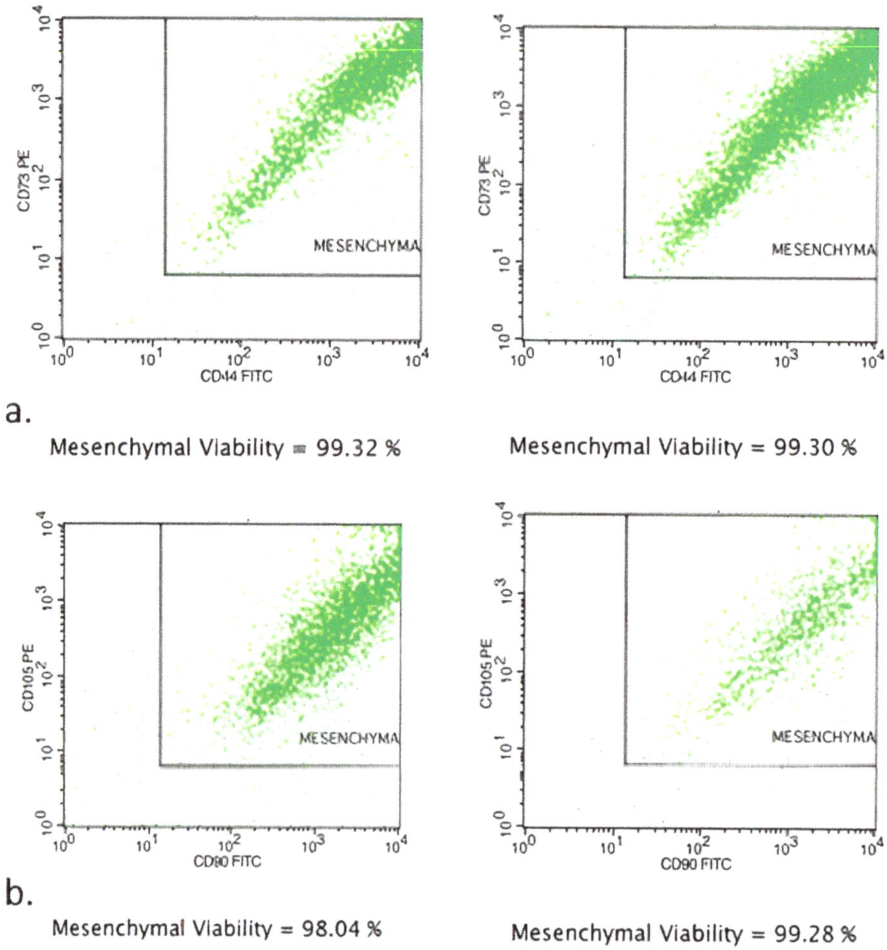

Figure 1. Flow cytometric analysis of MSCs characterized by the expression of MSCs markers. (**a**) MSCs were positive for CD73 (96.19% expression) and CD44 (97.31% expression). (**b**) MSCs were positive for CD90 (96.98% expression) and CD105 (92.46% expression).

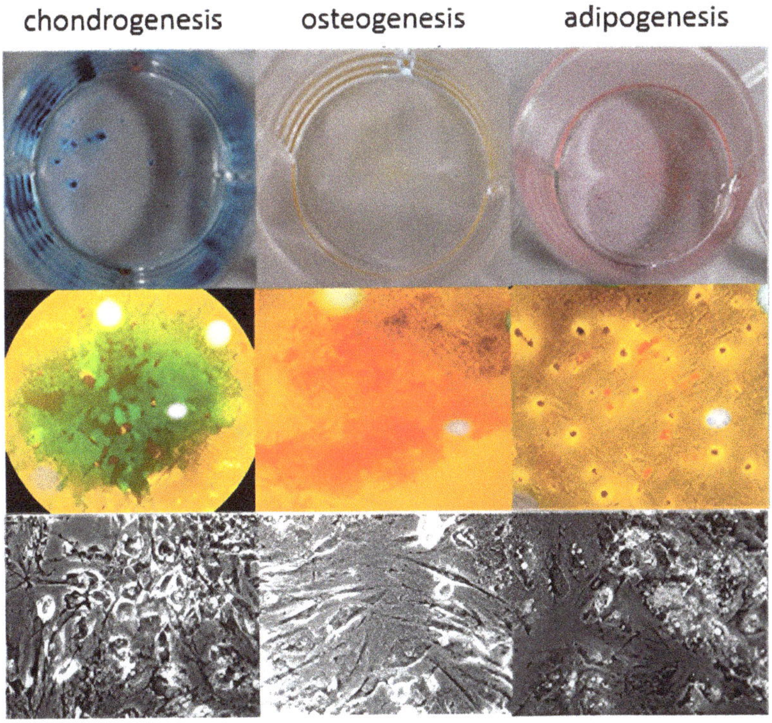

Figure 2. Tri-lineage differentiation (cartilage, bone and adipose tissue) potential of MSCs after 10 days of culture in differentiation mediums. This figure shows that the MSCs used in our study had a significant potential to differentiate and be appropriate for use.

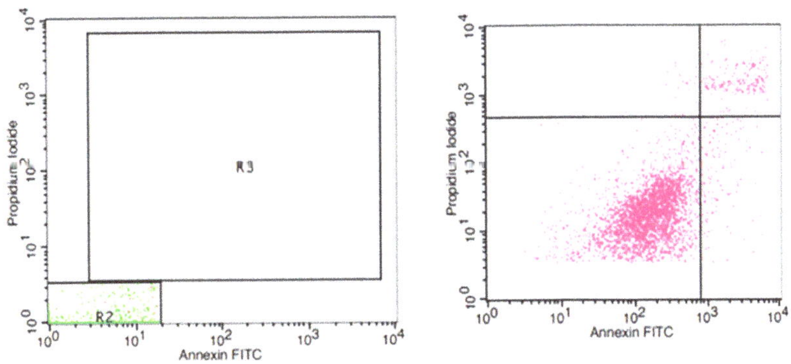

X Parameter: Annexin FITC (Log)
Y Parameter: Propidium Iodide (Log)
Quad Location: 806, 470

Quad	% Gated	X Geo Mean	Y Mean	Y Geo Mean
UL	0.62	430.32	1473.00	1310.93
UR	5.74	2913.28	1777.30	1595.10
LL	89.58	146.06	25.80	17.32
LR	4.07	1421.05	117.10	60.77

Figure 3. Representative results of flow cytometry for MSCs' viability after thawing.

2.4. Experimental Colitis

Experimental colitis was induced via transrectal administration of TNBS (Sigma-Aldrich, St. Louis, MO, USA). A solution of 5 mg TNBS dissolved in 0.5 mL 40% ethanol was prepared to be administered to all animals of groups 2 to 5. Under light ether anesthesia, a PE-50 cannula (8 cm long) was inserted into the colon via the anus, and a 0.25 mL of the above solution (40% ethanol containing 5 mg TNBS) was instilled into the lumen of the colon. Solution diffusion to the proximal colon and prevention of expulsion was performed by placing the animal in reverse position and holding the cannula intrarectally for one minute. All animals were assessed daily for clinical signs of colitis: presence of wet feces in the anal area, loose stools or diarrhea, bleeding per rectum, altered behavior, weight loss and piloerection. This procedure led to similar degrees of colitis. However, in order to avoid bias, the degree of colitis had been previously standardized via primary experiments using several dilutions of TNBS and ethanol and assessing the following parameters upon autopsy (no:0 and yes:1): 10% loss of body weight (0 or 1); wet anus, soft stool, or empty colon (0 or 1); anal bleeding/occult blood (0 or 1); macroscopic ulcers present (0 or 1); and death (0 or 1). To standardize experiments, a score of at least 2 to 3 degrees (score 2 or 3) was decided to be appropriate in order to avoid animal deaths and facilitate comparisons between groups. Also, all included animals should present macroscopic findings of colitis in the surgical specimen (Figure 4). Therefore, all animals having colitis of different degrees at autopsy were discarded and replaced by new ones for the comparisons. In total, 6 animals needed to be replaced for the final comparisons.

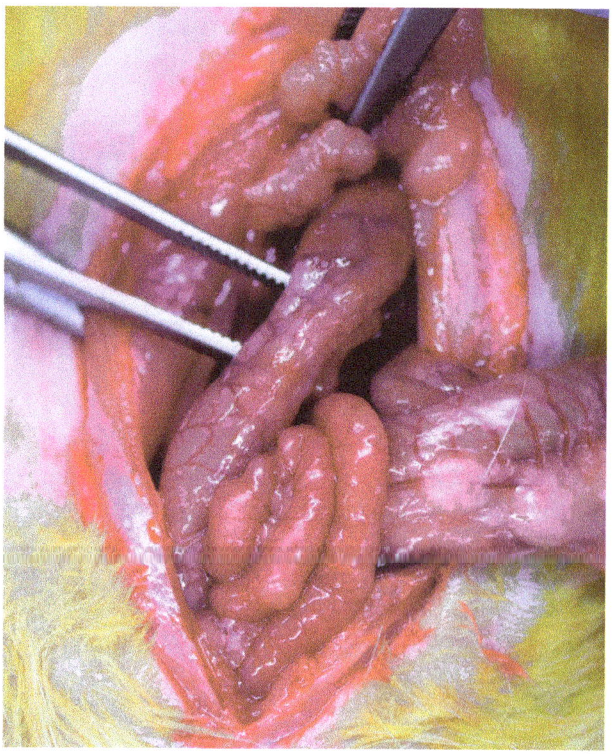

Figure 4. Intraoperative findings of macroscopic colitis. Forceps indicate a large bowel segment that presents signs of acute inflammation: hyperemia, induration, loose adhesions to the surrounding organs and edema.

2.5. Surgical Procedure

Rats were anaesthetized via intraperitoneal injection of ketamine hydrochloride (Ketalar®) and xylazine (Rompun®) at a dose of 50 mg/kg and 5 mg/kg, respectively. All surgical interventions were performed by the same surgeon (GG). Postoperative analgesia was achieved via intraperitoneal injection of paracetamol at a dose of 500 mg/kg. Following a midline laparotomy, a segmental colectomy 1 cm in length was performed on the inflamed area of the colon at approximately 3 cm's distance from the anus, as measured via insertion of an intrarectal catheter. The colon was sharply divided by knife, and immediately a 500 μL volume of PRP, MSCs or PRP+MSCs was injected submucosally at a depth of about 1 mm at 4 symmetrical sites in the intestinal wall of both intestinal stumps by making use of a fine (insulin injection) needle. Following that, anastomosis was performed via standard procedures using 8 single sutures of 6-0 Prolene stitches. The abdominal cavity was washed with normal saline and surgically closed. All animals received one dose of ciprofloxacin 500 mg/kg, metronidazole 500 mg/kg and paracetamol 500 mL/kg, intraperitoneally.

2.6. Autopsy—Macroscopic Examination

On day seven, all animals were sacrificed via neck dislocation, and the abdominal cavity was reopened and examined by two independent observer surgeons blinded to the interventions. Intraperitoneal adhesions, anastomotic leaks, collections, abscesses, inflammation or damages in surrounding organs were assessed and documented. Anastomotic leak was declared (or suspected) if free bowel content was noted in the abdominal cavity, or any presence of abscess or extensive adhesions in the perianastomotic area. All animals experiencing complications were included in the analysis.

2.7. Anastomotic Bursting Pressure (ABP) Measurement

A 4-cm piece of colon containing anastomosis in the middle was connected to a classical sphygmomanometer using a 3-way connector and a drip tube while the other end of the colon was tightly ligated. The colon was dived into a beaker filled with normal saline, and air was pumped into the 3-way entrance of the tube with a slow rate of 5 cc/min via use of a syringe pump. Bursting pressure was recorded at the time that the first air bubbles appeared at the site of anastomosis. Following this, the colon anastomotic site, which was defined as 0.5 cm bilaterally from the anastomotic line, was longitudinally divided into fragments for further evaluations. A portion was fixed in formalin for histology, and another portion was weighted and snap-frozen in liquid nitrogen for collagen measurements.

2.8. Histologic Examination

All colon specimens were fixed in formalin and embedded in paraffin. Hematoxylin-eosin stained sections were evaluated by two blinded pathologists without any knowledge of the groups. The specimens were evaluated for fibroblast cell concentration/density, neovascularization, inflammatory cell infiltration and anastomotic area epithelialization. The histopathological results of the groups were assessed according to the Phillips et al. scale [20]. Each of the aforementioned parameters was rated on a scale from 0 to 4: 0: None, 1: Slight increase, 2: Moderate infiltration, 3: Dense infiltration and 4: Confluent cells or fibers. For the assessment of epithelialization, a 0 to 3 scale was used: absent (zero points), incomplete cubic (one point), normal cubic (two points), or normal glandular (three points) [21].

2.9. Hydroxyproline Assessment

Tissues were initially weighed and homogenized mechanically via grinding using mortar and pestle and several cycles of freezing/thawing of the tissues in liquid nitrogen. For the assay, high-temperature glass tubes were used. Test samples were analyzed at a concentration of 100 μg/mL, and successive dilutions of a collagen solution (Achille's tendon, Sigma-Aldrich) were used for the preparation of a standard curve. Test samples/standards were firstly hydrolyzed via autoclaving for 20 min at 120 °C in NaOH (10.125 N). The pH of the samples/standards was subsequently regulated at 6–7 by adding HCl solution (8 N), followed by induction of hydroxyproline oxidation via incubation for 25 min at room temperature in a T-Chloramine solution (0.056 M in 10% isopropanol and 90% acetate-citrate buffer pH 6.5). The chromophore was then developed with the addition of Ehrlich's solution (1 M) and incubation for 20 min at 65 °C. The absorbance of a reddish complex was measured at 550 nm using a spectrophotometer. The absorbance values were plotted against the concentrations of standards, and the concentration of hydroxyproline in sample tissues was determined from the standard curve in μg/mL.

2.10. Statistical Analysis

The G*Power statistical software (Faul, Erdfelder, Lang, & Buchner, 2007, version 3.1.9.6) was used to calculate the sample size. A strong consideration of reduction principle from the 3Rs (replacement, reduction and refinement domains of animals used in research) took place. Data from a previously published animal study was used. An effect size of 0.69, five groups of animals, power of the test 80% and a significance level of $p < 0.05$ indicated a total number of 35 animals [22,23]. The histopathological values were expressed with median, first and third quadrantile. The anastomotic burst pressure and tissue hydroxyproline levels were presented with mean and standard deviations. Overall comparisons between groups for each of the histopathologic domain (inflammatory cell infiltration, angiogenesis, fibroblast activity and anastomotic area epithelialization), tissue hydroxyproline and anastomotic bursting pressure was performed with the Kruskal–Wallis test. When statistically significant differences were found, an unpaired, two-sided Mann–Whitney U test was performed to assess which of the individual groups presented statistically significant differences. A value of $p < 0.05$ was considered to be statistically significant.

3. Results

3.1. Autopsy

All animals presented clinical findings of colitis that included diarrhea, piloerection and reduced mobility. No mortality was noted throughout the study. Immediate or delayed immunoreactions reactions were not observed. No collections, free fluid or abscesses were detected. A few postoperative complications were detected: abdominal wound dehiscence (1/35 in MSCs group), anastomotic leak (2/35 in colitis control and MSCs group) and ileus (1/35 in colitis control group). The anastomotic leak was suspected to be due to dense adhesions around the anastomosis in two animals as mentioned above. In all other animals, anastomoses were intact without any dense adhesions.

3.2. APB

All anastomoses were subjected to APB measurement. In two cases, dense adhesions were observed around the anastomotic site. These two specimens were transferred into the ABP measuring devise en bloc, along with their adhesions. This was to keep the anastomosis intact while measuring the ABP. These samples exhibited very low ABP compared to the mean (65 and 80 mmHg), obviously due to leakage. All other anastomoses did not present any suspicion of perforation. The mean ± SD values of the anastomotic burst pressures were: 145.71 ± 62.14 (Group 1), 92.85 ± 77.82 (Group 2), 181.42 ± 99.57 (Group 3), 194.28 ± 132.39 (Group 4) and 288.57 ± 108.69 (Group 5) (Table 1). Animals treated with PRP+MSCs presented significantly higher ABPs compared to the normal (p = 0.0477) and colitis (p = 0.0104) control groups. The APB in the remaining group combinations did not reveal any statistical difference (Figure 5).

Table 1. Summary of the histopathological results. Numbers for the histopathological markers are presented in median (first quartile, third quartile) and for ABP (anastomotic bursting pressure) and tissue hydroxyproline in mean ± SD. Asterisk (*) indicates statistically significant differences.

Group	Inflammatory Cell Infiltration	Angiogenesis	Fibroblast Density	Epithelialization	ABP (mmHg)	Tissue Hydroxyproline (μg/mL)
Normal Control	3 (3, 4)	1 (1, 1) *	2 (1, 4)	1 (0, 1)	145.71 ± 62.14 *	109.14 ± 125.05
Colitis Control	4 (3, 4)	1 (1, 1) *	1 (0, 1)	0 (0, 1) *	92.85 ± 77.82 *	63.3 ± 72.29 *
MSCs	3 (3, 4)	1 (0, 1)	2 (1, 2)	1 (1, 2) *	181.42 ± 99.57	158.38 ± 168.17
PRP	4 (3, 4)	1 (0, 1)	2 (1, 3)	1 (0, 1)	194.28 ± 132.39	387.71 ± 275.55 *
PRP and MSCs	2 (2, 3)	2 (1, 2) *	2 (2, 3)	2 (1, 2) *	288.57 ± 108.69 *	457.95 ± 307.08 *

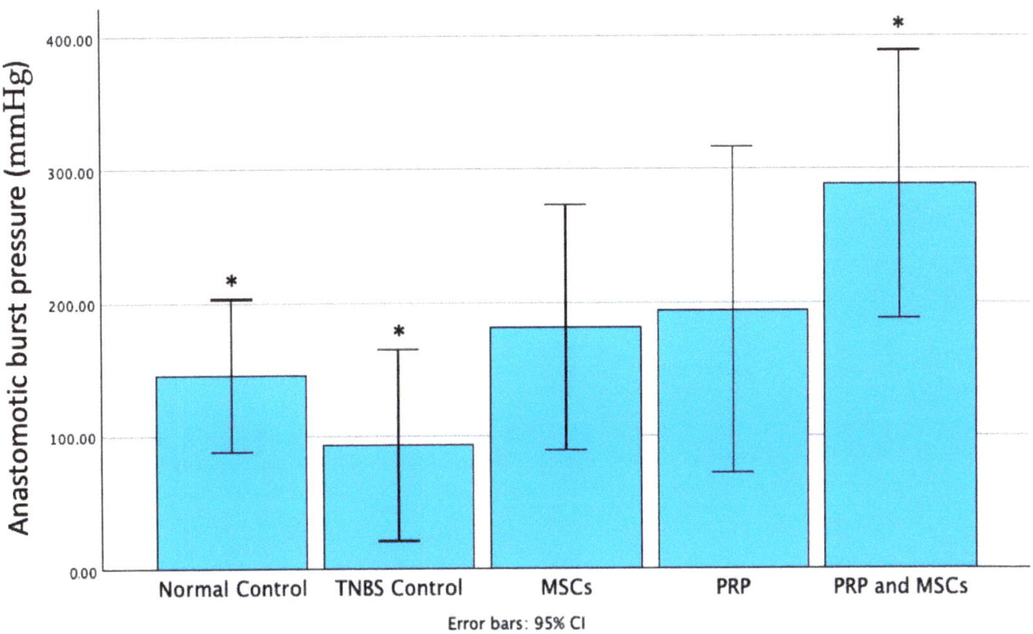

Figure 5. ABP calculation. PRP+MSCs present a statistically significant increased ABP over the TNBS control. Differences between normal control MSCs, PRP and combination of PRP and MSCs are not significant. Data presented as mean ± SD with the 95% confidence interval. Asterisk (*) indicates statistically significant differences.

3.3. Histopathological Examination

The inflammatory cell infiltration, angiogenesis, fibroblast density and anastomotic area epithelialization were assessed. Specifically, regarding the inflammatory cell infiltration, despite being lower in the PRP+MSCs group, no statistically significant difference was found when compared to the rest of the groups ($p = 0.0832$). Angiogenesis was significantly higher in PRP+MSCs group compared to the TNBS colitis ($p = 0.0073$) and normal control ($p = 0.0214$) group. Epithelialization scores were significantly higher in the PRP alone ($p = 0.348$) and PRP+MSCs ($p = 0.0182$) group compared to the colitis control. Fibroblast activity was higher in the PRP group alone and PRP+MSCs group; however, no statistically significant differences were found in all group comparisons ($p = 0.1118$). Table 1 summarizes the median (first quartile, third quartile) of the histopathological scores as well as the tissue hydroxyproline and ABP mean ± standard deviation values. The plots in Figure 6 show the differences between controls and PRP, MSCs and PRP+MSCs groups. Histopathological photos presenting the improved healing of PRP+MSCs compared to the colitis control group is shown in Figure 7A,B.

3.4. Hydroxyproline Levels

Hydroxyproline levels reflect collagen production in healing tissues. The mean ± SD values for the tissue hydroxyproline levels were as follows: 109.14 ± 125.05 (Group 1), 63.3 ± 72.29 (Group 2), 158.38 ± 168.17 (Group 3), 387.71 ± 275.55 (Group 4), 457.95 ± 307.08 (Group 5). Our results revealed a statistically significant difference between groups. More specifically, tissue hydroxyproline was significantly higher in the MSCs (p = 0.03) and PRP+MSCs (p = 0.0151) groups compared to the TNBS colitis control group. Tissue hydroxyproline in the remaining group combinations did not reveal any statistical difference. Therefore, there is collagen upregulation in the MSCs and much more in the PRP+MSCs group (Figure 8).

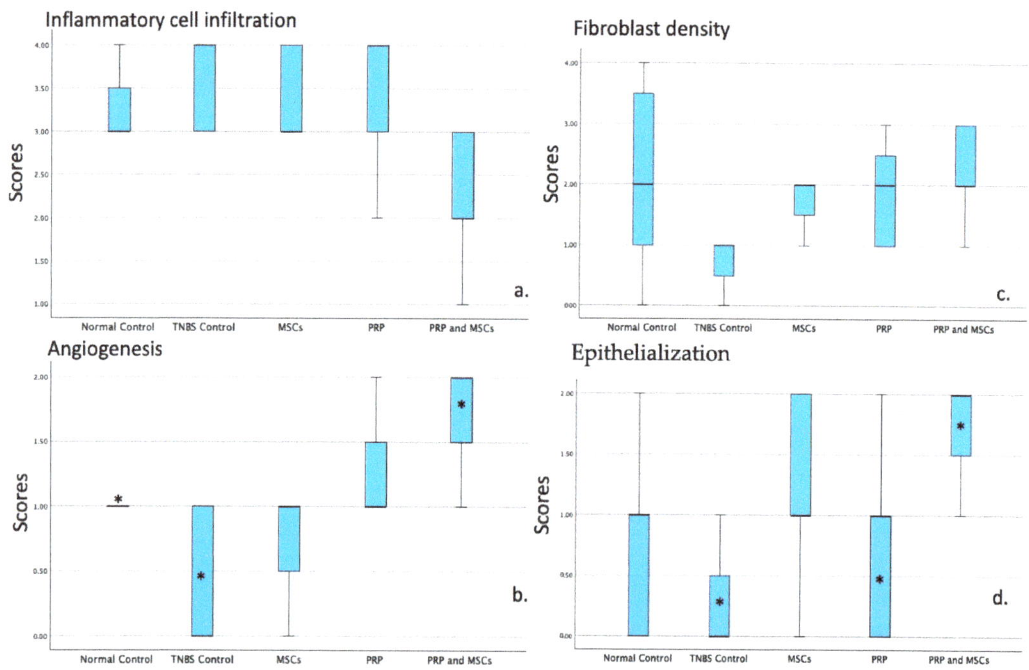

Figure 6. Histopathology box plots of the inflammatory cell infiltration (**a**), angiogenesis (**b**), fibroblast density (**c**) and anastomotic area epithelialization (**d**). Each of the aforementioned parameters scored on a scale from 0 to 4: 0: None, 1: Slight increase, 2: Moderate infiltration, 3: Dense infiltration and 4: Confluent cells or fibers. For the assessment of epithelialization a 0 to 3 scale was used: absent (zero points), incomplete cubic (one point), normal cubic (two points), or normal glandular (three points). Values were presented as median, first, third quartile and 95% confidence interval. Asterisk (*) indicates statistically significant differences.

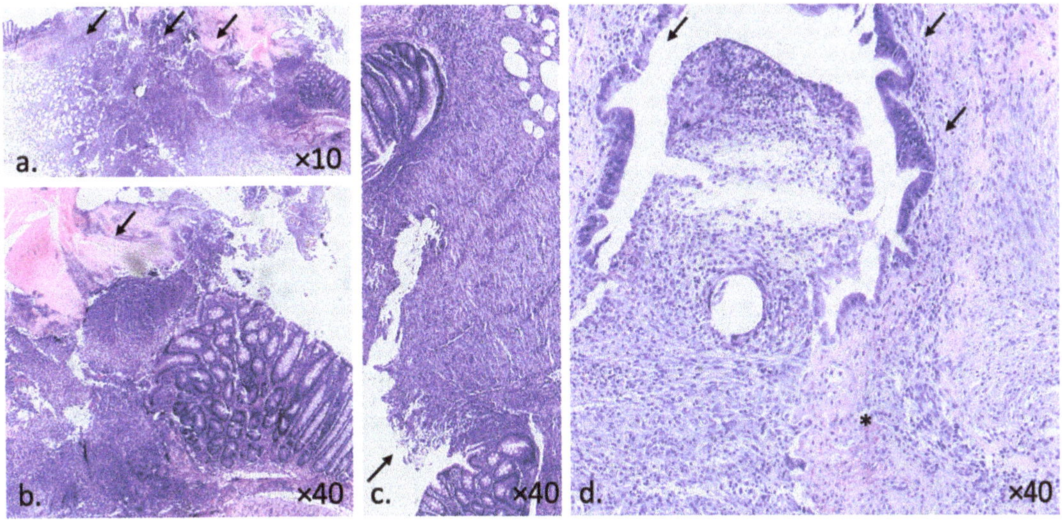

(**A**)

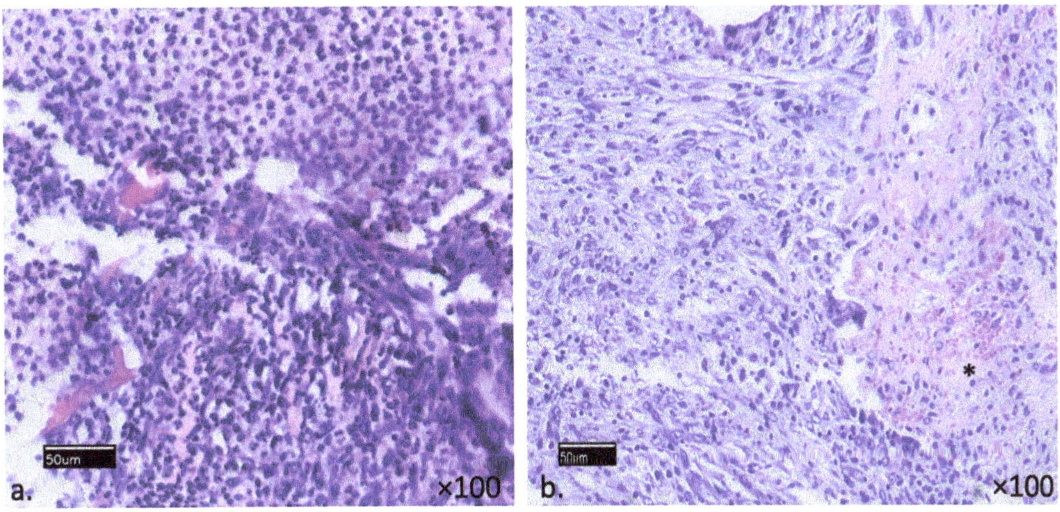

(**B**)

Figure 7. (**A**) Histopathological appearance of colonic anastomotic site in colitis control group (**a**,**b**) and PRP+MSCs treatment group (**c**,**d**). Arrows indicate the anastomotic line area. Colitis control group shows increased anastomotic area distance and absence of epithelialization (**a**), also friable anastomotic area tissue with solely inflammatory cell infiltration without evidence of fibrous tissue formation (**b**). In PRP+MSCs group there is prominent collagen deposition along with inflammatory cell infiltration (**c**), evidence of muscular tissue formation (*) and progenitor epithelial cells starts to cover the anastomotic area along with underlying dense capillaries ((**d**), arrows). (**B**) Greater magnitude (×100) of the colitis control and PRP+MSCs group at the anastomotic line area. (**a**) Colitis control group: dense inflammatory cell infiltration with up to 30% necrosis. (**b**) PRP+MSCs group: less inflammatory cell deposition, evidence of neoangiogenesis with visible small vessel structures (*) with up to 5% necrosis.

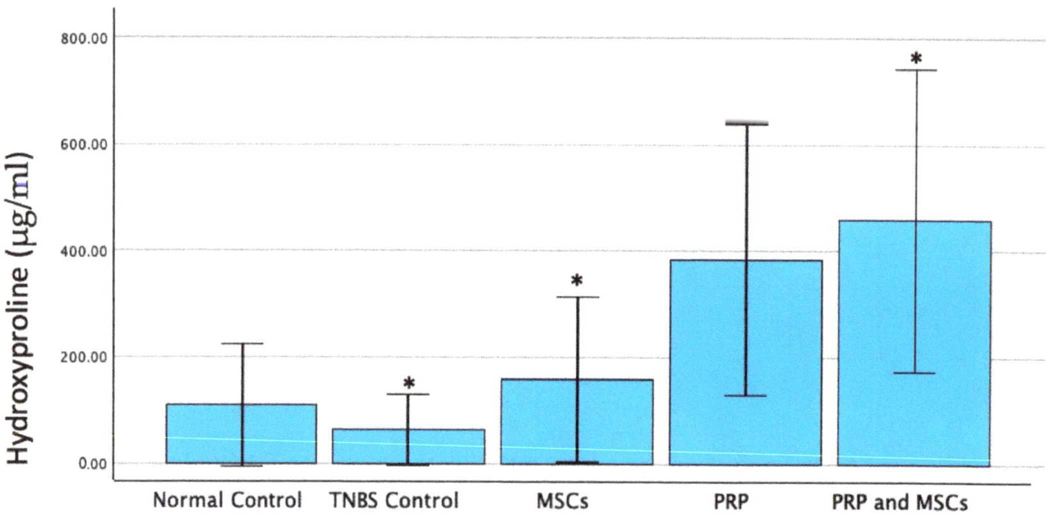

Figure 8. Tissue hydroxyproline levels. Tissue hydroxyproline was significantly higher in the MSCs group (p = 0.03) and PRP+MSCs group (p = 0.0151) compared to the TNBS colitis control group. Tissue hydroxyproline in the remaining group combinations did not reveal any statistical difference. Asterisk (*) indicates statistically significant differences.

4. Discussion

To the best of our knowledge, this is the first study investigating the effect of the combined administration of PRP and adipose tissue-derived MSCs on inflammatory bowel anastomoses after the establishment of experimental colitis in rats. Our results indicate that the infiltration of the enteric stumps with a combination of these two agents gives an impressive boost in the enteric wall healing even on inflammatory bowel. This result may be due to enhanced collagen deposition, as indicated via the significantly increased tissue hydroxyproline levels in the PRP+MSCs group samples. Additionally, the significantly increased neovascularization and epithelialization at the anastomotic line of PRP+MSCs group may also have contributed to the intestinal healing improvement. PRP alone or MSCs alone showed improved anastomotic area healing compared to colitis controls, however, that was not statistically significant; therefore, these two agents need to be applied together in order to exert their synergistic effect. Apparently, the PRP environment, which is rich in nutrients and growth factors, may act as a medium for MSCs to efficiently heal the anastomotic site. Furthermore, reduced inflammatory cell infiltration was detected; thus, PRP+MSCs may also mediate certain anti-inflammatory actions, as has been previously described by others [8,9].

The healing process seems to differ in different parts of the gastrointestinal tract like the stomach and small and large bowel [24,25]. Previous studies have shown that colonic anastomosis has a slower rate of healing compared to the ones performed in the ileum. Small bowel anastomosis reaches its normal strength in about 4 weeks, in contrast to large bowel anastomosis, which, even after 4 months, gains only 75% of its strength [26,27]. This fact also potentiates the need to find agents that could enhance the colonic anastomotic healing, especially in pathologic conditions like ischemia or inflammation, where the healing process is impaired. The healing process of bowel anastomosis is a series of overlapping events. Three classic stages have been described: the exudative, the proliferative and the remodeling phase [6]. Systemic inflammatory cells like neutrophils, macrophages, platelets and fibroblasts exert their role at the exudative phase. Platelets are responsible for the cessation of further blood loss from the bowel wound edge, but not exclusively. Platelets secrete multiple growth factors as well. These factors induce cell migration, proliferation, extracellular matrix synthesis and angiogenesis. Other factors that promote angiogenesis include hypoxia, EGF, endothelin 1, TNF-a, interleukin 1b, monocyte chemotactic protein-1 (MCP-1) and macrophage inflammatory protein (MIP-1a) [28]. After two to fourteen days, the proliferative phase is characterized by cellular proliferation, angiogenesis and reproduction of extracellular matrix. At this stage, macrophages that reside at the anastomotic area serve as growth factor-secreting cells, which promote the formation of the epithelium. In addition, on the fourth postoperative day, fibroblasts are the most prominent cells at the anastomotic site. The presence of PDGF, TGF-b, FGF and IGF-I mostly regulate fibroblast activity. It is quite clear that both MSCs and PRP, with their derivative factors, participate actively in all stages of the intestinal wound healing process [29]. Our study results indicate that PRP+MSCs led to reduced inflammatory cell infiltration, although non-significant. The improved healing in of the PRP+MSCs group may have been assisted by reduced inflammatory cell infiltration. Previous studies have shown that MSCs may reduce inflammatory cell infiltration in tissues and may facilitate the healing process [30,31].

Application of MSCs or PRP have been separately tested in bowel anastomoses in previously experimental animal studies. Administration of stem cells in the anastomotic area in animal models with ischemia or radiation injury report a lower occurrence of anastomotic leaks [32]. Alvarenga et al. reported that adipose tissue-derived MSCs in a TNBS colitis rat model significantly reduce certain tissue inflammatory cells (CD4+ T cells, macrophages) and certain tissue inflammatory cytokines (IL-17, TNF-a and IFN-γ) [33]. A systematic review on the effect of PRP in bowel anastomosis included 16 animal studies. Their results indicate that PRP is safe to administer and provides a significant benefit in animals with peritonitis or post-intraperitoneal chemotherapy application. However, compared with normal controls, PRP did not provide any significant benefit over the bowel anastomosis healing process [18]. These findings are keeping in line with our results where the PRP+MSCs group provided a significant benefit in bowel anastomosis healing over the colitis control group, however when compared with normal controls, no significant changes were observed. Another example of clinical application of MSCs include the Crohn's colitis perianal fistulas. An early clinical trial in 2005 showed that adipose-derived MSCs showed an up to 60% healing rate of perianal fistulas [34]. Panes et al., in their randomized clinical trial of Darvadstrocel (Alofisel®), one of the first commercially available adult MSCs suspension, reported its effectiveness and safety of use for treating complex perianal Crohn's fistulas [35]. Considering the facts (firstly, that MSCs are commercially available; secondly, that PRP is easily produced via a simple venipuncture/centrifugation and thirdly, the outcomes of our study), future clinical studies of PRP+MSCs in humans could be seriously considered.

Co-administration of MSCs and PRP has also been investigated in several experimental and clinical settings of other pathologies. Ebrahim et al. showed that their combined administration significantly improved epithelialization, collagen deposition and angiogenesis in wound healing of diabetic foot ulcers [36]. In a preclinical model of osteoarthritis, there was improved healing of the articular cartilage with MSCs preconditioned in PRP. Combination of MSCs and PRP seems to augment collagen and proteoglycan contents in the knee joint [37]. A clinical study by Gentile et al. concluded that when adipose tissue-derived MSCs were mixed with PRP for breast fillings, the overlying post-radiotherapy damaged skin was improved [38]. These findings are consistent with the results of our study, since the application of PRP+MSCs led to improved epithelialization and neovascularization at the anastomotic site.

Collagen formation is possibly the main factor leading to stronger bowel anastomoses. It has been reported that the submucosa layer of the bowel wall plays a significant role in supporting the tensile strength of bowel anastomoses. In the submucosa layer the collagen type I predominates, followed by types III and IV. Type I and III collagens are the predominant ones in the granulation and scar tissue following bowel anastomosis [39]. The significant increase in the tissue hydroxyproline levels suggest a considerable increase on collagen production at the anastomotic site which was further higher in the PRP+MSCs group rather than in the MSCs alone group.

Neovascularization is another critical factor for efficient healing. Our study shows that the PRP+MSCs increases vascular formation at the anastomotic area. Surgeons know very well that impaired blood supply to enteric stumps leads to healing failure and anastomotic disruption, therefore they always care to leave intact as much vasculature as possible during dissection. Several studies exist to support the value of neovascularization, which seems to be upregulated by MSCs. Chen et al. showed that MSCs preconditioned with PRP exhibited improved neovascularization in ischemic rat hind limb models [40].

In the clinical setting, gastrointestinal anastomoses are an everyday routine for the general surgeon, and traditionally, there are certain technical rules for good results without complications, which are basic for any surgery trainee. The stumps must be well mobilized to permit free peristalsis, should not be inflammatory (if there is any site of inflammation, it should be excised), well vascularized to permit free blood supply, and finally good and meticulous technique in suturing the layers of the gastrointestinal tract should be followed. This should also be accompanied by efficient parenteral nutritive support, use of drains and patience of both the patient and the surgeon. Nevertheless, whatever measures are taken, often anastomoses are disrupted, and that can be sometimes disastrous, especially at sites where direct vision and manipulations are not easy, and the use of staplers is the only solution, such as in the esophageal or rectal stumps; surgeons can never be sure of the technical efficiency of anastomoses. In fact, the percentage of anastomotic leaks is as high as 17.5% in pancreaticojejunal anastomoses, 14.6% in esophagojejunal anastomoses and up to 17% in ileocecal anastomoses [4–6]. These numbers are even higher in immunocompromised or malnourished patients and even more so in emergency and infective/inflammatory settings. Consequently, the results of such complications are very often detrimental, leading to mediastinitis or peritonitis, severe sepsis, systemic inflammatory response syndrome, reoperations, extra enterectomies, new anastomoses and vice versa [41].

Therefore, finding an agent that improves intestinal wound healing and allows for the safe performance of bowel anastomoses, thus avoiding a stoma, was one of the targets of this study. To avoid risky anastomoses, surgeons have the option of reverting stomas whenever applicable. Colostomies and ileostomies have been the gold standard in aid of anastomoses. Stomas have saved lives of many patients, especially in emergency settings. Hartmann's procedure is the most frequent operation on the colon in all departments of surgery around the globe for obstructive ileus of the left colon, either neoplastic or inflammatory. Transverse colostomies and reverting ileostomies are performed in similar pathologies of the transverse and right colon respectively. Prophylactic stomas, created centrally, are another solution for those surgeons who dare to perform anastomoses in risky cases. However, except the surgeon, not all others are happy with the stoma solution. Patients have difficulty in accepting them, their families often have difficulty supporting patients, and nursing staff are often unhappy in approaching patients. The total cost of hospital stay, re-admissions, patient training, reoperations, disposable materials for stomas etc. seems to be tremendous [42]

Therefore, in surgical practice whenever any inflammatory environment, such as peritonitis, colitis, enteritis, etc., is present, anastomoses should be avoided. Stoma creation, either permanent or prophylactic, is absolutely necessary. On the other hand, and very unfortunately, inflammatory bowel diseases such as ulcerative colitis and Crohn's disease have been constantly increasing over the past decades in the Western world [43]. Similarly, and even more so, diverticulitis and its complications have been dramatically increasing even in the young population due to extensive stress, fast food remedies and lack of fiber in modern Western dietary habits [44]. Moreover, ischemic colitis is also increasing [45]. Very lately, pseudomembranous colitis has seemed to start a new chapter of severe inflammatory and life-threatening septic situations due to antibiotic overuse [46]. Finally, post-radiation colitis is also a new problem due to therapeutic cancer remedies in the pelvis [47]. Although stomas are a safe classical solution in such cases, in the new era of surgery, a more sophisticated way should be applied in order to strengthen gastrointestinal anastomoses. MSC and PRP co-administration seem to give hope for such a target, as the results of our study suggest. This can be further explained. On the cellular level, multipotent progenitor cells seem to somehow recognize the needs of the tissue where they are placed; they possibly mediate local inflammation decrease via cytokine regulation, and they transform into fibroblasts to produce the correct collagen fibers, while they promote neovascularization and epithelialization of the tissue to make it appropriate [48]. The exact mediators for such a behavior need to be further investigated.

In our experiments, we used heterogenic adipose tissue-derived MSCs. Whether this category of stem cells is appropriate for application in anastomoses is not clear. Nevertheless, it is a feasible approach that can be easily generalized, and it is safe as well. Neither did we observe any significantly increased complications such as stenoses, ileus, immunoreactions or rejection. Besides, as previously commented, heterologous adipose tissue MSCs have already been commercialized in vials and used for the treatment of Crohn's fistulas in patients, with encouraging results [49]. If they work well for fistulas why not work well for anastomoses either, they could easily be mixed with PRP prepared from the same patient and be applied even in the emergency settings. Additionally, autologous stem cells from the patient could also be prepared if there is at least 1 month time before any scheduled operation [50]. Recently, a rapid adipose tissue MSCs isolation method (isolation of stem cells within 8 h after fat removal) has been described [51]. Is there a need for that or not, that also remains to be investigated. Possibly, heterologous stem cells are safe enough for this purpose, and we do not need to try further. A clinical study incorporating many of these questions is in need of approval by our institution, and hopefully it will soon be scheduled in multiple settings. In our experiments, we simply injected the mixture of MSCs and PRP into the intestinal wall with fine needle insulin syringes at four sites of the intestinal stump periphery. This is the simplest way to do this; however, we can think of more efficient forms of administration. For example, absorbing material for sutures, or biodegradable circular membranes infused with the active solution, or even manufacturing staplers to deliver the active solution along with stapling would be excellent ideas to make surgery safe and effective for our purpose for a strong intestinal anastomosis.

5. Conclusions

In conclusion, our study supports the use of MSCs+PRP in inflammatory bowel anastomoses, with excellent results in strengthening anastomotic healing with increased collagen deposition, neovascularization and improved epithelialization at the anastomotic site. The translation of this study to the clinical practice requires further research in clinical and pre-clinical settings to establish the safety and effectiveness of MSC and PRP co-administration in gastrointestinal anastomoses in humans.

Author Contributions: Conceptualization, K.P.; methodology, K.P., M.P., N.S., G.K. (Georgios Koliakos) and T.E.P.; software, G.G., V.G., G.K. (Georgios Koimtzis), N.S. and E.T.P.; validation, K.P., T.E.P., I.G. and T.E.P.; stem cell investigation, A.N.; formal analysis, G.G. and A.N.; investigation, G.G. and V.G.; data curation, G.G.; resources, G.G. and V.G.; writing—original draft, G.G.; writing—review and editing, K.P.; supervision, K.P., M.P. and T.E.P.; funding acquisition, G.G.; pathology investigation, C.N.; project administration, K.P., M.P. and G.K. (Georgios Koliakos); resources, K.P. and G.K. (Georgios Koliakos); visualization, G.G., V.G. and G.K. (Georgios Koimtzis). All authors have read and agreed to the published version of the manuscript.

Funding: This research received no external funding.

Institutional Review Board Statement: The animal study protocol was approved by the Institutional Review Board (protocol code EL-54-BIOexp-10 and date of approval 11 September 2023).

Informed Consent Statement: Not applicable.

Data Availability Statement: The data presented in this study are available on request from the corresponding author (accurately indicate status).

Acknowledgments: This review is part of a Ph.D. thesis research project, taking place at the School of Medicine, Aristotle University, Thessaloniki, Greece. Special thanks to Ioannis Taitzoglou, School of Veterinary Medicine, Faculty of Health Sciences, Aristotle University of Thessaloniki, Thessaloniki for his support.

Conflicts of Interest: Author Niti A., employer and Koliakos G., director of Biohellenika Biotechnology Company report no conflict of interest. The remaining authors declare that the research was conducted in the absence of any commercial or financial relationships that could be construed as a potential conflict of interest. The Biohellenika Biotechnology Company had no role in the design of the study; in the collection, analyses, or interpretation of data; in the writing of the manuscript, or in the decision to publish the results.

References

1. Kang, C.Y.; Halabi, W.J.; Chaudhry, O.O.; Nguyen, V.; Pigazzi, A.; Carmichael, J.C.; Mills, S.; Stamos, M.J. Risk factors for anastomotic leakage after anterior resection for rectal cancer. *JAMA Surg.* **2013**, *148*, 65–71. [CrossRef] [PubMed]
2. Hyman, N.; Manchester, T.L.; Osler, T.; Burns, B.; Cataldo, P.A. Anastomotic leaks after intestinal anastomosis: It's later than you think. *Ann. Surg.* **2007**, *245*, 254–258. [CrossRef] [PubMed]
3. Yauw, S.T.K.; Wever, K.E.; Hoesseini, A.; Ritskes-Hoitinga, M.; van Goor, H. Systematic review of experimental studies on intestinal anastomosis. *Br. J. Surg.* **2015**, *102*, 726–734. [CrossRef]
4. Azagra, J.S.; Makkai-Popa, S.T.; Pascotto, B.; Arru, L.; De Blasi, V.; Ramia, J.M.; Ibanez-Aguirre, F.J.; Goergen, M. Laparoscopic pancreaticojejunal anastomosis using knotless barbed absorbable sutures are simple, safe and effective: An experience with 34 procedures. *Laparosc. Surg.* **2020**, *4*, 27. [CrossRef]
5. Makuuchi, R.; Irino, T.; Tanizawa, Y.; Bando, E.; Kawamura, T.; Terashima, M. Esophagojejunal anastomotic leakage following gastrectomy for gastric cancer. *Surg. Today* **2019**, *49*, 187–196. [CrossRef] [PubMed]
6. Garofalo, E.; Lucarini, A.; Flashman, K.G.; Celentano, V. A positive proximal resection margin is associated with anastomotic complications following primary ileocaecal resection for Crohn's disease. *Int. J. Colorectal. Dis.* **2019**, *34*, 1585–1590. [CrossRef]
7. Malik, T.; Lee, M.J.; Harikrishnan, A.B. The incidence of stoma related morbidity—A systematic review of randomised controlled trials. *Ann. R Coll. Surg. Engl.* **2018**, *100*, 501–508. [CrossRef]
8. Van de Putte, D.; Demarquay, C.; Van Daele, E.; Van Daele, E.; Moussa, L.; Vanhove, C.; Benderitter, M.; Ceelen, W.; Pattyn, P.; and Mathieu, N. Adipose-Derived Mesenchymal Stromal Cells Improve the Healing of Colonic Anastomoses Following High Dose of Irradiation Through Anti-Inflammatory and Angiogenic Processes. *Cell Transpl.* **2017**, *26*, 1919–1930. [CrossRef]
9. Sorrell, J.M.; Caplan, A.I. Topical delivery of mesenchymal stem cells and their function in wounds. *Stem. Cell Res Ther.* **2010**, *1*, 1–6. [CrossRef]
10. Wu, Y.; Chen, L.; Scott, P.G.; Tredget, E.E. Mesenchymal stem cells enhance wound healing through differentiation and angiogenesis. *Stem Cells* **2007**, *25*, 2648–2659. [CrossRef]
11. Mazini, L.; Rochette, L.; Admou, B.; Amal, S.; Malka, G. Hopes and limits of adipose-derived stem cells (ADSCs) and mesenchymal stem cells (MSCs) in wound healing. *Int. J. Mol. Sci.* **2020**, *21*, 1306. [CrossRef] [PubMed]
12. Trevor, L.V.; Riches-Suman, K.; Mahajan, A.L.; Thornton, M.J. Adipose tissue: A source of stem cells with potential for regenerative therapies for wound healing. *J. Clin. Med.* **2020**, *9*, 2161. [CrossRef] [PubMed]
13. Altman, A.M.; Yan, Y.; Matthias, N.; Bai, X.; Rios, C.; Mathur, A.; Song, Y.-H.; Alt, E.U. IFATS Collection: Human Adipose-Derived Stem Cells Seeded on a Silk Fibroin-Chitosan Scaffold Enhance Wound Repair in a Murine Soft Tissue Injury Model. *Stem Cells* **2009**, *27*, 250–258. [CrossRef] [PubMed]
14. Hu, L.; Wang, J.; Zhou, X.; Xiong, Z.; Zhao, J.; Yu, R.; Huang, F.; Zhang, H.; Chen, L. Exosomes derived from human adipose mensenchymal stem cells accelerates cutaneous wound healing via optimizing the characteristics of fibroblasts. *Sci. Rep.* **2016**, *6*, 32993. [CrossRef] [PubMed]
15. Özçay, N.; Özdemir, H.; Besim, H. Role of platelet-rich fibrin on intestinal anastomosis wound healing in a rat. *Biomed. Mater.* **2018**, *13*, 045006.
16. Estcourt, L.J.; Malouf, R.; Hopewell, S.; Trivella, M.; Doree, C.; Stanworth, S.J.; Murphy, M.F. Pathogen- reduced platelets for the prevention of bleeding. *Cochrane Database Syst. Rev.* **2017**, *7*, CD009072. [CrossRef]
17. Mio, T.; Adachi, Y.; Romberger, D.J.; Ertl, R.F.; Rennard, S.I. Regulation of fibroblast proliferation in three- dimensional collagen gel matrix. *In Vitro Cell Dev. Biol. Anim.* **1996**, *32*, 427–433. [CrossRef]
18. Geropoulos, G.; Psarras, K.; Giannis, D.; Martzivanou, E.C.; Papaioannou, M.; Kakos, C.D.; Pavlidis, E.T.; Symeonidis, N.; Koliakos, G.; Pavlidis, T.E. Platelet rich plasma effectiveness in bowel anastomoses: A systematic review. *World J. Gastrointest. Surg.* **2021**, *13*, 1736. [CrossRef]
19. Antoniou, E.; Margonis, G.A.; Angelou, A.; Pikouli, A.; Argiri, P.; Karavokyros, I.; Papalois, A.; Pikoulis, E. The TNBS-induced colitis animal model: An overview. *Ann. Med. Surg.* **2016**, *11*, 9–15. [CrossRef]

20. Philips, J.D.; King, C.S.; Fonkalsrud, E.W.; Zeng, H.; Dindar, H. Effect of cronic corticosteroid and vitamin A on the healing of intestinal anastomoses. *Am. J. Surg.* **1992**, *163*, 71–77. [CrossRef]
21. Verhofstad, M.H.; Lange, W.P.; van der Laak, J.A.; Verhofstad, A.A.; Hendriks, T. Microscopic analysis of anastomotic healing in the intestine of normal and diabetic rats. *Dis. Colon Rectum.* **2001**, *44*, 423–431. [CrossRef] [PubMed]
22. Alakuş, H.; Göksu, M.; Erten, S. Early enteral nutrition with L-glutamine improves anastomotic healing in rats administered hyperthermic intraperitoneal chemotherapy with cisplatin and 5-FU. *J. Surg. Med.* **2021**, *5*, 848–852. [CrossRef]
23. Cohen, J.; A power primer. In Methodological Issues and Strategies in Clinical Research; Kazdin, A.E., Ed.; 2016, 279–284. Available online: https://psycnet.apa.org/record/2015-32022-018 (accessed on 24 December 2023).
24. Thompson, S.K.; Chang, E.Y.; Jobe, B.A. Clinical review: Healing in gastrointestinal anastomoses, part I. *Microsurg. Off. J. Int. Microsurg. Soc. Eur. Fed. Soc. Microsurg.* **2006**, *26*, 131–136. [CrossRef] [PubMed]
25. Enestvedt, C.K.; Thompson, S.K.; Chang, E.Y.; Jobe, B.A. Clinical review: Healing in gastrointestinal anastomoses, part II. *Microsurg. Off. J. Int. Microsurg. Soc. Eur. Fed. Soc. Microsurg.* **2006**, *26*, 137–143. [CrossRef] [PubMed]
26. Mast, B.A. Healing in other tissues. *Surg. Clin. North. Am.* **1997**, *77*, 529–547. [CrossRef]
27. Martens, M.F.; Hendriks, T. Postoperative changes in collagen synthesis in intestinal anastomoses of the rat: Differences between small and large bowel. *Gut* **1991**, *32*, 1482–1487. [CrossRef]
28. Radulescu, A.; Zhang, H.Y.; Chen, C.L.; Chen, Y.; Zhou, Y.; Yu, X.; Otabor, I.; Olson, J.K.; Besner, G.E. Heparin-binding EGF- like growth factor promotes intestinal anastomotic healing. *J. Surg. Res.* **2011**, *171*, 540–550. [CrossRef]
29. Rijcken, E.; Sachs, L.; Fuchs, T.; Spiegel, H.U.; Neumann, P.A. Growth factors and gastrointestinal anastomotic healing. *J. Surg. Res.* **2014**, *187*, 202–210. [CrossRef]
30. Feng, B.; Feng, X.; Yu, Y.; Xu, H.; Ye, Q.; Hu, R.; Fang, X.; Gao, F.; Wu, J.; Pan, Q.; et al. Mesenchymal stem cells shift the pro-inflammatory phenotype of neutrophils to ameliorate acute lung injury. *Stem Cell Res Ther.* **2023**, *14*, 197. [CrossRef]
31. Huh, J.W.; Kim, W.Y.; Park, Y.Y.; Lim, C.M.; Koh, Y.; Kim, M.J.; Hong, S.B. Anti-inflammatory role of mesenchymal stem cells in an acute lung injury mouse model. *Acute Crit. Care.* **2018**, *33*, 154–161. [CrossRef]
32. Gaitanidis, A.; Kandilogiannakis, L.; Filidou, E.; Tsaroucha, A.; Kolios, G.; Pitiakoudis, M. Stem Cell Therapies for Gastrointestinal Anastomotic Healing: A Systematic Review and Meta-Analysis on Results from Animal Studies. *Eur. Surg. Res.* **2022**, *63*, 173–181. [CrossRef] [PubMed]
33. Alvarenga, V., Jr.; da Silva, P.T.; Bonfá, N.D.; Pêgo, B.; Nanini, H.; Bernardazzi, C.; Madi, K.; da Cruz, W.B.; Castelo-Branco, M.T.; de Souza, H.S.; et al. Protective effect of adipose tissue–derived mesenchymal stromal cells in an experimental model of high-risk colonic anastomosis. *Surgery* **2019**, *166*, 914–925. [CrossRef]
34. García-Olmo, D.; García-Arranz, M.; Herreros, D.; Pascual, I.; Peiro, C.; Rodríguez- Montes, J.A. A phase I clinical trial of the treatment of Crohn's fistula by adipose mesenchymal stem cell transplantation. *Dis. Colon. Rectum.* **2005**, *48*, 1416–1423. [CrossRef] [PubMed]
35. Panés, J.; García-Olmo, D.; Van Assche, G.; Colombel, J.F.; Reinisch, W.; Baumgart, D.C.; Dignass, A.; Nachury, M.; Ferrante, M.; Kazemi-Shirazi, L.; et al. Expanded allogeneic adipose-derived mesenchymal stem cells (Cx601) for complex perianal fistulas in Crohn's disease: A phase 3 randomised, double-blind controlled trial. *Lancet* **2016**, *388*, 1281–1290. [CrossRef]
36. Ebrahim, N.; Dessouky, A.A.; Mostafa, O.; Hassouna, A.; Yousef, M.M.; Seleem, Y.; El Gebaly, E.A.; Allam, M.M.; Farid, A.S.; Saffaf, B.A.; et al. Adipose mesenchymal stem cells combined with platelet-rich plasma accelerate diabetic wound healing by modulating the Notch pathway. *Stem. Cell Res. Ther.* **2021**, *12*, 1–24. [CrossRef] [PubMed]
37. Ahmad, M.R.; Badar, W.; Ullah Khan, M.A.; Mahmood, A.; Latif, N.; Iqbal, T.; Khan Assir, M.Z.; Sleem, M.A. Combination of preconditioned adipose-derived mesenchymal stem cells and platelet-rich plasma improves the repair of osteoarthritis in rat. *Regen Med.* **2020**, *15*, 2285–2295. [CrossRef] [PubMed]
38. Gentile, P.; Pasquali, C.D.; Bocchini, I.; Floris, M.; Eleonora, T.; Fiaschetti, V. Breast Reconstruction with Autologous Fat Graft Mixed with Platelet-Rich Plasma. *Surg. Innov.* **2013**, *20*, 370–376. [CrossRef]
39. Witte, M.B.; Barbul, A. Repair of full-thickness bowel injury. *Crit. Care. Med.* **2003**, *31*, S538–S546. [CrossRef]
40. Chen, C.F.; Liao, H.T. Platelet-rich plasma enhances adipose-derived stem cell-mediated angiogenesis in a mouse ischemic hindlimb model. *World J. Stem. Cells.* **2018**, *10*, 212. [CrossRef]
41. Girard, E.; Messager, M.; Sauvanet, A.; Benoist, S.; Piessen, G.; Mabrut, J.Y.; Mariette, C. Anastomotic leakage after gastrointestinal surgery: Diagnosis and management. *J. Visc. Surg.* **2014**, *151*, 441–450. [CrossRef]
42. Kawai, M.; Sakamoto, K.; Honjo, K.; Okazawa, Y.; Takahashi, R.; Kawano, S.; Munakata, S.; Sugimoto, K.; Ishiyama, S.; Takahashi, M.; et al. Benefits and risks of diverting stoma creation during rectal cancer surgery. *Ann. Coloproctol.* **2022**. *Epub ahead of print*. [CrossRef] [PubMed]
43. Buie, M.J.; Quan, J.; Windsor, J.W.; Coward, S.; Hansen, T.M.; King, J.A.; Kotze, P.G.; Gearry, R.B.; Ng, S.C.; Mak, J.W.Y.; et al. Global Hospitalization Trends for Crohn's Disease and Ulcerative Colitis in the 21st Century: A Systematic Review with Temporal Analyses. *Clin. Gastroenterol. Hepatol.* **2023**, *21*, 2211–2221. [CrossRef]
44. Strate, L.L.; Morris, A.M. Epidemiology, Pathophysiology, and Treatment of Diverticulitis. *Gastroenterology* **2019**, *156*, 1282–1298. [CrossRef]
45. Cai, W.; Zhu, J.; Hu, D. Clinical features and risk factors for ischemic colitis in young and middle-aged patients. *Acta. Gastroenterol. Belg.* **2022**, *85*, 283–290. [CrossRef] [PubMed]

46. Selvaraj, V.; Alsamman, M.A. Antibiotic-Associated Diarrhea Beyond C. Difficile: A Scoping Review. *Brown Hosp. Med.* **2022**, 2. [CrossRef]
47. Fan, J.; Lin, B.; Fan, M.; Niu, T.; Gao, F.; Tan, B.; Du, X. Research progress on the mechanism of radiation enteritis. *Front. Oncol.* **2022**, *12*, 888962. [CrossRef]
48. Gentile, P.; Scioli, M.G.; Bielli, A.; De Angelis, B.; De Sio, C.; De Fazio, D.; Ceccarelli, G.; Trivisonno, A.; Orlandi, A.; Cervelli, V.; et al. Platelet-rich plasma and micrografts enriched with autologous human follicle mesenchymal stem cells improve hair re-growth in androgenetic alopecia. biomolecular pathway analysis and clinical evaluation. *Biomedicines* **2019**, *7*, 27. [CrossRef]
49. Cao, Y.; Su, Q.; Zhang, B.; Shen, F.; Li, S. Efficacy of stem cells therapy for Crohn's fistula: A meta-analysis and systematic review. *Stem Cell Res. Ther.* **2021**, *12*, 1–11. [CrossRef]
50. Mushahary, D.; Spittler, A.; Kasper, C.; Weber, V.; Charwat, V. Isolation, cultivation, and characterization of human mesenchymal stem cells. *Cytom. Part A* **2018**, *93*, 19–31. [CrossRef]
51. Francis, M.P.; Sachs, P.C.; Elmore, L.W.; Holt, S.E. Isolating adipose-derived mesenchymal stem cells from lipoaspirate blood and saline fraction. *Organogenesis* **2010**, *6*, 11–14. [CrossRef]

Journal of *Personalized Medicine*

Article

Endoscopic Transpapillary Stenting for Malignant Hilar Biliary Stricture: Side-by-Side Placement versus Partial Stent-in-Stent Placement

Koji Takahashi [1,2,*], Hiroshi Ohyama [1], Yuichi Takiguchi [2], Motoyasu Kan [1], Mayu Ouchi [1], Hiroki Nagashima [1], Izumi Ohno [1,2] and Naoya Kato [1]

1 Department of Gastroenterology, Graduate School of Medicine, Chiba University, Chiba 260-8670, Japan
2 Department of Medical Oncology, Graduate School of Medicine, Chiba University, Chiba 260-8670, Japan
* Correspondence: takahashi.koji@chiba-u.jp; Tel.: +81-43-226-2083

Abstract: Background/Aims: Endoscopic uncovered metal stent (UMS) placement has been widely performed for unresectable hilar malignant biliary stricture (UHMBS). Two stenting methods are used for the two bile duct branches: side-by-side placement (SBS) and partial stent-in-stent placement (PSIS). However, it remains controversial whether SBS or PSIS is superior. This study aimed to compare SBS and PSIS in UHMBS cases with UMS placement in two branches of the IHD. Methods: This retrospective study included 89 cases of UHMBS treated with UMS placement through the SBS or PSIS technique using endoscopic retrograde cholangiopancreatography at our institution. Patients were divided into two groups, SBS ($n = 64$) and PSIS ($n = 25$), and compared. Results: Clinical success was achieved in 79.7% and 80.0% in the SBS and PSIS groups, respectively ($p = 0.97$). The adverse event rate was 20.3% and 12.0% in the SBS and PSIS groups, respectively ($p = 0.36$). The recurrent biliary obstruction (RBO) rate was 32.8% and 28.0% in the SBS and PSIS groups, respectively ($p = 0.66$). The median cumulative time to RBO was 224 and 178 days in the SBS and PSIS groups, respectively ($p = 0.52$). The median procedure time was 43 and 62 min in the SBS and PSIS groups, respectively, which was significantly longer in the PSIS group ($p = 0.014$). Conclusions: No significant differences were noted in the clinical success rate, adverse event rate, time to RBO, or overall survival between the SBS and PSIS groups, other than the significantly longer procedure time in the PSIS group.

Keywords: endoscopic retrograde cholangiopancreatography; hilar malignant biliary stricture; partial stent-in-stent; side-by-side; stent

1. Background/Aims

Hilar malignant biliary stricture (HMBS) is caused by cholangiocarcinoma, gallbladder carcinoma, hepatocellular carcinoma, metastatic liver tumors, or hilar lymph node metastases from various cancers. HMBSs induce high serum bilirubin concentrations owing to cholestasis, which is called obstructive jaundice. Obstructive jaundice affects the biliary tree, hepatic cells, and liver functions. Additionally, the loss of bile in the gut disrupts the intestinal mucosal barrier, which increases the absorption of endotoxins from the intestine [1]. The symptoms of obstructive jaundice include itching, loss of appetite, and weight loss. Effective biliary drainage is required to improve the quality of life of HMBS patients. Although percutaneous biliary drainage and surgical biliary drainage are also available, endoscopic biliary drainage is recommended because it is less invasive. Endoscopic biliary drainage includes transpapillary drainage using endoscopic retrograde cholangiopancreatography (ERCP) and transgastrointestinal drainage using endoscopic ultrasonography. Unless there is a special reason, such as duodenal obstruction or post-operative gastrointestinal reconstruction, transpapillary drainage using ERCP is the first choice. Transpapillary drainage by ERCP involves endoscopic biliary stenting and endoscopic nasobiliary drainage. In unresectable HMBS (UHMBS), endoscopic biliary stenting is usually performed. Two types of biliary stents are used for endoscopic biliary stenting: plastic stents and metal stents. Several studies have shown that metal stents outperform patients with unresectable UHMBS in terms of patency and cost efficiency [2,3]. Thus, endoscopic uncovered metal stent (UMS) placement has been widely performed for UHMBS. Previously, unilateral UMS placement was the mainstream treatment for biliary drainage in UHMBS [4]. However, biliary drainage of >50% of the liver volume was reported to be associated with effective drainage for UHMBS in several studies [5,6]. Furthermore, a recent randomized controlled trial revealed better stent patency with bilateral UMS placement than with unilateral UMS placement for UHMBS [7]. Therefore, bilateral UMS placement is typically performed for UHMBS.

Regarding bilateral UMS placement using the ERCP, two stenting methods are used: side-by-side placement (SBS) and partial stent-in-stent placement (PSIS). SBS is a procedure in which two guidewires are placed in two branches of the intrahepatic bile duct (IHD), and then two stent deliveries are inserted and deployed sequentially. The routes of the two UMSs are independent of each other. Meanwhile, PSIS is a procedure in which the first stent is deployed, followed by another stent inserted through the mesh of the first stent and deployed (Figure 1). As a procedure, the PSIS is more complex.

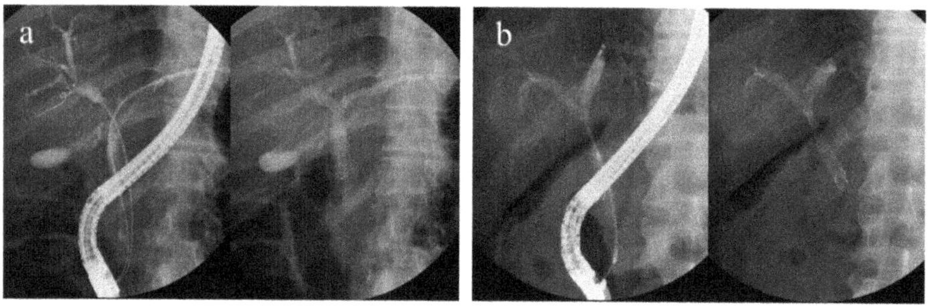

Figure 1. (**a**) Side-by-side placement and (**b**) partial stent-in-stent placement.

Several reports have compared SBS and PSIS, but no conclusion has been drawn as to which is superior, and it remains controversial. Most previous reports indicate that there is no difference in performance between SBS and PSIS; however, they have been from high-volume centers, and their results might not be universal. This is because the majority of procedures may have been performed only by expert endoscopists. At our institution, there are many opportunities for trainees to perform endoscopic treatment under the supervision of experts; therefore, we decided to examine features of SBS and PSIS, including the endoscopist's proficiency. This study aimed to compare SBS and PSIS in UHMBS cases with UMS placement in two branches of the IHD.

2. Materials and Methods

2.1. Study Design

This retrospective study was conducted at a single center. A total of 89 patients with UHMBS treated with UMS placement in two branches of the IHD using the ERCP technique between April 2006 and December 2022 were studied from the database of Chiba University Hospital. HMBS was diagnosed based on computed tomography (CT) and histopathological examination. In cases where histopathological malignant findings were unclear or histopathological examination was difficult, the diagnosis was made if a typical CT image could be confirmed. The resectability was judged comprehensively from the findings, including CT images and cholangiography. The exclusion criteria were as follows: (1) patients aged <20 years; (2) patients with percutaneous transhepatic biliary drainage continued even after UMS placement; (3) patients with Bismuth type I; (4) patients with biliary tract reconstruction; (5) patients with stent placements in three or more branches of the IHD in a single ERCP session; (5) patients with unclear background and treatment information; and (6) patients judged as inappropriate by the investigators. This study was approved by the ethics committee of our institution. Written informed consent for the procedure was obtained from all patients.

Participants were divided into two groups: the SBS group and the PSIS group. Baseline characteristics and clinical outcomes were obtained from the patients' medical records and compared between the two groups. The baseline characteristics included age, sex, the proportion of direct UMS placement at the first ERCP session, pre-ERCP serum total bilirubin level, pre-ERCP serum albumin level, Bismuth type, extrahepatic bile duct diameter in the tumor-free area before stent placement, the causes of malignant biliary obstruction, the proportion of above the papilla stent placement, endoscopist proficiency, and the proportion of chemotherapy after UMS placement. The clinical outcomes included procedure time, clinical success rate, adverse event rate, recurrent biliary obstruction (RBO) rate, cumulative time to RBO (TRBO) in effective drainage cases, re-intervention rate, technical success rate of the first re-intervention, procedure time of the first re-intervention, and overall survival.

2.2. Definitions

Clinical success, RBO, and adverse events were defined according to the Tokyo criteria 2014 [8]. Clinical success was defined as a decrease in the serum total bilirubin level to <50% or <2.0 mg/dL within 14 days of stent placement, without additional biliary drainage. RBO was defined as a composite endpoint, including stent occlusion and migration. TRBO refers to the time from stent placement to RBO. Deaths without RBO were treated as censored at the time of death. Patients lost to follow-up without RBO were treated as censored at the time of the final follow-up. Stent occlusion was defined as the occurrence of jaundice with cholestasis and evidence of bile duct dilation on imaging or endoscopy. Procedure time was defined as the time interval between insertion of the endoscope into the mouth and its removal. The extrahepatic bile duct diameter in the tumor-free area was measured on cholangiography during ERCP. In re-intervention, technical success was defined as additional stent placement or balloon sweep for a UMS judged to be obstructed by CT images.

2.3. Techniques

Placement of the UMS was performed transpapillary using the ERCP technique. Prior to UMS placement, CT was performed, and the biliary drainage area was planned based on the liver volume in all cases. Prophylactic intravenous antibiotics were administered before the procedure. ERCP was performed using an oblique-viewing endoscope (JF-260V, TJF-260V, and TJF-Q290V; Olympus, Tokyo, Japan). In the absence of contraindications, carbon dioxide insufflation was used during ERCP. All patients underwent intravenous sedation. Sodium meglumine amidotrizoate was used as a contrast medium. An endoscope was inserted orally to reach the duodenal papilla, and an ERCP catheter (PR-104Q-1; Olympus, Tokyo, Japan. MTW; ABIS, Hyogo, Japan. SwingTip; Olympus, Tokyo, Japan) was inserted into the bile duct. After cholangiography and identifying the site of biliary stenosis with a contrast medium, guidewires (VisiGlide; Olympus, Tokyo, Japan. VisiGlide 2; Olympus, Tokyo, Japan. M-Through; ASAHI INTECC, Aichi, Japan. EndoSelector; Boston Scientific, Marlborough, MA, USA) were placed in two branches of the IHD. Subsequently, UMSs (Zilver 635 Biliary Stent; Cook Medical, Bloomington, IN, USA. X-Suit NIR; Olympus, Tokyo, Japan. WallFlex; Boston Scientific, Marlborough, MA, USA. Niti-S D-type; Century Medical, Tokyo, Japan. BileRush; Piolax, Yokohama, Japan. JOSTENT; Zeon Medical, Tokyo, Japan. Zeo Stent V; Zeon Medical, Tokyo, Japan. YABUSAME; Kaneka, Osaka, Japan.) were deployed in two branches of the IHD. For SBS, after the insertion of the guidewires into the two branches of the IHD, two stent deliveries were inserted into the IHDs and sequentially deployed. For PSIS, the first stent was inserted into one IHD after the insertion of guidewires into the two IHDs. Subsequently, after deploying the first stent, the guidewire was passed through the mesh of the first stent into another IHD. The second stent was deployed through the mesh of the first stent. All procedures were performed by experts on ERCP (≥10 years of ERCP experience) or by trainees (<10 years of ERCP experience) under the supervision of experts. If the operator changed during the procedure, the physician who had operated the endoscope for a long time was defined as the operator of the procedure.

2.4. Statistical Analysis

Data were presented as median with interquartile range or number with a percentage. For the univariate analysis, the Mann–Whitney U test was used to compare continuous variables, whereas Pearson's Chi-squared test was used to compare categorical variables. Cumulative TRBO and overall survival were estimated using Kaplan–Meier analysis, and Kaplan–Meier curves were compared using the log-rank test. Statistical significance was set at $p < 0.05$. All statistical analyses were performed using Bell Curve for Excel (Social Survey Research Information Co., Ltd., Tokyo, Japan).

3. Results

The age of the study participants ranged from 36 to 90 years, with a median of 71 (64–79) years. Of the 89 patients, 64 underwent SBS, and 25 underwent PSIS. All patients underwent endoscopic sphincterotomy before UMS placement.

Patient characteristics of the two groups are presented in Table 1. The median age was 71 (66–79) and 71 (63–79) years in the SBS and PSIS groups, respectively ($p = 0.84$). The proportion of men in the SBS and PSIS groups was 67.2% and 64.0%, respectively ($p = 0.78$). The proportions of direct UMS placement at the first ERCP session were 15.6% and 28.0% in the SBS and PSIS groups, respectively ($p = 0.18$). The median pre-ERCP serum total bilirubin level was 4.8 (1.4–8.4) and 8.1 (2.1–11.6) mg/dL in the SBS and PSIS groups, respectively ($p = 0.12$). The median pre-ERCP serum albumin level was 2.7 (2.4–3.2) and 3.0 (2.5–3.7) mg/dL in the SBS and PSIS groups, respectively ($p = 0.17$). Regarding the Bismuth type, the proportion of type II was 15.6% and 8.0% in the SBS and PSIS groups, respectively ($p = 0.34$). The proportions of type IIIa were 20.3% and 44.0% in the SBS and PSIS groups, respectively, and significantly higher in the PSIS group ($p = 0.024$). The proportions of type IIIb were 15.6% and 20.0% in the SBS and PSIS groups, respectively ($p = 0.62$). The proportions of type IV were 48.4% and 28.0% in the SBS and PSIS groups, respectively ($p = 0.080$). The median extrahepatic bile duct diameter in the tumor-free area was 8.7 (7.2–9.9) and 6.6 (6.1–7.2) mm in the SBS and PSIS groups, respectively, significantly larger in the SBS group ($p < 0.01$). Regarding causes of malignant biliary obstruction, the proportion of hilar cholangiocarcinoma was 48.4% and 48.0% in the SBS and PSIS groups, respectively ($p = 0.97$). The proportion of gallbladder cancer in the SBS and PSIS groups was 17.2% and 28.0%, respectively ($p = 0.25$). The proportions of intrahepatic cholangiocarcinoma in the SBS and PSIS groups were 6.3% and 4.0%, respectively ($p = 0.68$). The proportions of hepatocellular carcinoma in the SBS and PSIS groups were 10.9% and 12.0%, respectively ($p = 0.89$). The proportion of metastatic liver tumors in the SBS and PSIS groups was 10.9% and 8.0%, respectively ($p = 0.68$). The proportions of hilar lymph node metastases in the SBS and PSIS groups were 6.3% and 0%, respectively ($p = 0.20$). The proportion of patients above-the-papilla stent placement in the SBS and PSIS groups was 90.6% and 88.0%, respectively ($p = 0.71$). The proportions of expert performance in the SBS and PSIS groups were 20.3% and 48.0%, respectively, and significantly higher in the PSIS group ($p < 0.01$). The proportions of chemotherapy after UMS placement were 32.8% and 36.0% in the SBS and PSIS groups, respectively ($p = 0.78$). No significant differences were noted in terms of age, sex, the proportion of direct UMS placement at the first ERCP session, pre-ERCP serum total bilirubin level, pre-ERCP serum albumin level, the proportion of the causes of malignant biliary obstruction, the proportion of above the papilla stent placement, or the proportion of chemotherapy after UMS placement between the two groups.

Table 1. Patient characteristics of the two groups.

	SBS Group $n = 64$	PSIS Group $n = 25$	p-Value
Age, year, median (IQR)	71 (66–79)	71 (63–79)	0.84
Sex, man, n (%)	43 (67.2%)	16 (64.0%)	0.78
Direct UMS placement at the first ERCP session, n (%)	10 (15.6%)	7 (28.0%)	0.18
Pre-ERCP serum total bilirubin level, mg/dL, median (IQR)	4.8 (1.4–8.4)	8.1 (2.1–11.6)	0.12
Pre-ERCP serum albumin level, mg/dL, median (IQR)	2.7 (2.4–3.2)	3.0 (2.5–3.7)	0.17
Bismuth type, n (%)			
Type II	10 (15.6%)	2 (8.0%)	0.34
Type IIIa	13 (20.3%)	11 (44.0%)	0.024
Type IIIb	10 (15.6%)	5 (20.0%)	0.62
Type IV	31 (48.4%)	7 (28.0%)	0.080
Extrahepatic bile duct diameter in the tumor-free area before stent placement, mm, median (IQR)	8.7 (7.2–9.9)	6.6 (6.1–7.2)	<0.01
Causes of malignant biliary obstruction, n (%)			
Hilar cholangiocarcinoma	31 (48.4%)	12 (48.0%)	0.97
Gallbladder cancer	11 (17.2%)	7 (28.0%)	0.25
Intrahepatic cholangiocarcinoma	4 (6.3%)	1 (4.0%)	0.68
Hepatocellular carcinoma	7 (10.9%)	3 (12.0%)	0.89
Metastatic liver tumor	7 (10.9%)	2 (8.0%)	0.68
Hilar lymph nodes metastasis	4 (6.3%)	0	0.20
Above the papilla stent placement, n (%)	58 (90.6%)	22 (88.0%)	0.71
Operators, expert, n (%)	13 (20.3%)	12 (48.0%)	<0.01
Chemotherapy after UMS placement, n (%)	21 (32.8%)	9 (36.0%)	0.78

SBS, side-by-side placement; PSIS, partial stent-in-stent placement; IQR, interquartile range; UMS, uncovered metal stent; ERCP, endoscopic retrograde cholangiopancreatography.

Clinical outcomes in the SBS and PSIS groups are shown in Table 2. The median procedure time was 43 (28–53) and 62 (40–74) min in the SBS and PSIS groups, respectively, and significantly longer in the PSIS group than in the SBS group ($p = 0.014$). Clinical success was achieved in 79.7% and 80.0% in the SBS and PSIS groups, respectively ($p = 0.97$). The adverse event rate was 20.3% and 12.0% in the SBS and PSIS groups, respectively ($p = 0.36$). Regarding adverse events, the proportion of cholangitis in the SBS and PSIS groups was 7.8% and 4.0%, respectively ($p = 0.52$). The proportions of pancreatitis in the SBS and PSIS groups were 6.3% and 4.0%, respectively ($p = 0.68$). The proportions of liver abscesses in the SBS and PSIS groups were 3.1% and 0%, respectively ($p = 0.37$). The proportions of pneumonia in the SBS and PSIS groups were 1.6% and 4.0%, respectively ($p = 0.49$). The proportions of heart failure in the SBS and PSIS groups were 1.6% and 0%, respectively ($p = 0.53$).

The RBO rates in the SBS and PSIS groups were 32.8% and 28.0%, respectively ($p = 0.66$). Stent occlusion was the only cause of RBO, and there were no cases of stent migration. The median cumulative TRBO in the effective drainage cases was 224 and 178 days in the SBS and PSIS groups, respectively ($p = 0.52$) (Figure 2).

Table 2. Clinical outcomes of the two groups.

	SBS Group $n = 64$	PSIS Group $n = 25$	p-Value
Procedure time, minutes, median (IQR)	43 (28–53)	62 (40–74)	0.014
Clinical success, n (%)	51 (79.7%)	20 (80.0%)	0.97
Adverse events, n (%)	13 (20.3%)	3 (12.0%)	0.36
Cholangitis	5 (7.8%)	1 (4.0%)	0.52
Pancreatitis	4 (6.3%)	1 (4.0%)	0.68
Liver abscess	2 (3.1%)	0	0.37
Pneumonia	1 (1.6%)	1 (4.0%)	0.49
Heart failure	1 (1.6%)	0	0.53
RBO, n (%)	21 (32.8%)	7 (28.0%)	0.66
Cumulative TRBO in effective drainage cases, days, median (95% CI)	224 (91–357)	178 (74–282)	0.52
Re-intervention, n (%)	20 (31.2%)	7 (28.0%)	0.76
Technical success rate of the first re-intervention, n (%)	18 (90.0%)	7 (100%)	0.38
Procedure time of first re-intervention, min, median (IQR)	39 (30–70)	37 (33–55)	0.76
Overall survival, days, median (95% CI)	212 (105–319)	160 (83–237)	0.36

SBS, side-by-side placement; PSIS, partial stent-in-stent placement; IQR, interquartile range; CI, confidence interval; RBO, recurrent biliary obstruction; TRBO, time to recurrent biliary obstruction.

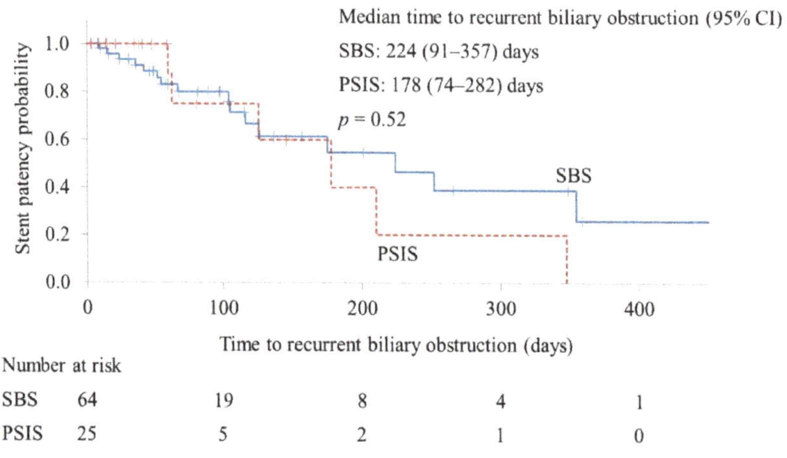

Figure 2. Kaplan–Meier curves of the time to recurrent biliary obstruction. CI, confidence interval; SBS, side-by-side placement, PSIS, partial stent-in-stent placement.

The re-intervention rates in the SBS and PSIS groups were 31.2% and 28.0%, respectively ($p = 0.76$). The technical success rates of the first re-intervention were 90.0% and 100% in the SBS and PSIS groups, respectively ($p = 0.38$). The median procedure time of the first re-intervention was 39 and 37 min in the SBS and PSIS groups, respectively ($p = 0.76$). The median overall survival was 212 and 160 days in the SBS and PSIS groups, respectively ($p = 0.36$) (Figure 3).

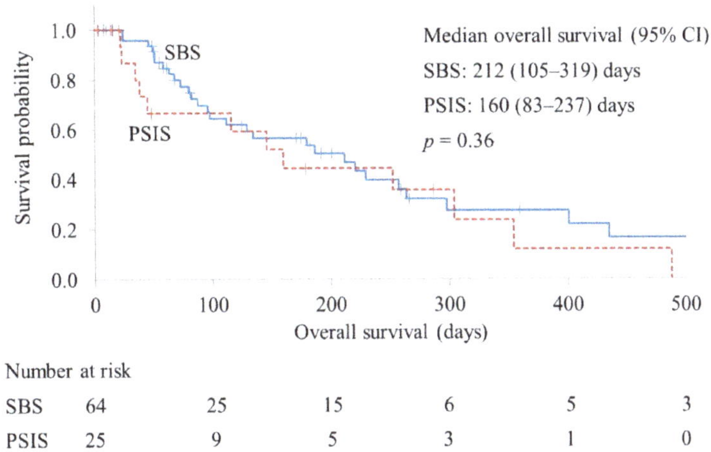

Figure 3. Kaplan–Meier curves of overall survival. CI, confidence interval; SBS, side-by-side placement; PSIS, partial stent-in-stent placement.

4. Discussion

In this study, we compared SBS and PSIS in UHMBS cases treated with UMS placement in two branches of the IHD and found that there was no significant difference in the clinical success rate, adverse event rate, RBO rate, cumulative TRBO in effective drainage cases, re-intervention rate, technical success rate of the first re-intervention, procedure time of the first re-intervention, or overall survival between the SBS and PSIS groups other than that the procedure time was significantly longer in the PSIS group, despite the higher rate of expert enforcement in PSIS compared to SBS. Adverse events included cholangitis, pancreatitis, liver abscess, pneumonia, and heart failure, none of which occurred disproportionately in either SBS or PSIS.

In this study, the rate of expert enforcement was significantly higher in PSIS than in SBS, probably because the procedure was more complex in PSIS, so there were more opportunities for experts to perform it. The reason for the predominance of Bismuth IIIa in PSIS is unclear. There is no set standard for the proper use of SBS and PSIS, and it depends on the policy of each institution. In PSIS, there is little concern regarding bile duct overdilation. Meanwhile, in SBS, the bile ducts are overextended due to the parallel insertion of the two stents, raising concerns such as portal vein obstruction. However, there were no such adverse events in this study.

Unilateral stenting was reported to be sufficient for effective biliary drainage in patients with UHMBS in two studies published in 2003 [4,9]. However, several reports have subsequently reported that drainage of >50% of the variable liver volume is an important drainage predictor and signals effective palliation in patients with UHMBS [5,6]. In recent years, several studies have reported the efficacy of multiple stenting for UHMBS [7,10–14]. To date, there are only five reports comparing SBS and PSIS, except for a meta-analysis. In 2012, Naitoh reported that deploying SBS resulted in a higher frequency of early and late adverse events than deploying PSIS placement. However, cumulative stent patency was prolonged in the SBS group in their single-center retrospective study (28 patients with SBS and 24 patients with PSIS) [15]. In 2012, Kim reported that adverse events, stent patency, and survival were not significantly different between the SBS and PSIS groups in a single-center retrospective study (19 patients with SBS and 22 patients with PSIS) [16]. In 2019, Lee reported that the efficacy of bilateral SIS and SBS placement was similar in terms of total adverse event rate, technical and clinical success, and stent patency in a randomized controlled trial (35 patients with SBS and 34 patients with PSIS) [17]. In 2020, Ishigaki reported that the clinical outcomes of the SBS and PSIS methods were comparable in patients with unresectable hilar malignant biliary obstruction in their multicenter retrospective study (24 patients with SBS and 40 patients with PSIS) [18]. In 2022, Iwai reported that the technical success rate, procedure duration, clinical success rate, adverse event rate, TRBO, and RBO rate were not significantly different between the SIS and SBS groups. However, endoscopic re-stenting after RBO was significantly more successful in the SBS group than in the SIS group in a single-center retrospective study (30 patients with SBS and 75 patients with PSIS) [19]. Few studies have examined the proficiency of endoscopists. In a retrospective report by Ishigaki, similar to this study, the proportion of experts performing PSIS was significantly higher than that performing SBS; however, in the study, there was no significant difference in the procedure time between SBS and PSIS [18].

In our study, procedure times were significantly longer in the PSIS group, despite the high percentage of procedures performed by expert endoscopists in the PSIS group. This is considered to be due to the fact that the procedure is more complex in PSIS than in SBS. In this study, there was a 19 min difference in the median procedure time between the SBS and PSIS groups. Few studies have investigated the relationship between the incidence of adverse events and procedure time in ERCP. In 2014, Mehta compared 177 ERCP procedures with <45 min to 118 ERCP procedures with >45 min and found no significant difference in the occurrence rates of adverse events [20]. Although not ERCP, in 2016, Kawanishi reported that a procedure time of 30 min or longer was a significant risk factor in the development of aspiration pneumonia after endoscopic hemostasis for upper gastrointestinal bleeding [21]. In 2022, Park reported that a procedure time of 80 min or longer in gastric endoscopic submucosal dissection is a risk factor for the onset of aspiration pneumonia after the procedure [22]. Although there are no clear data for ERCP, there is a concern that the risk of aspiration pneumonia increases with prolonged procedure time in ERCP. In particular, in patients at a high risk of aspiration pneumonia, such as the elderly or those with poor performance status, it may be preferable to choose SBS over PSIS. However, with a median difference of 19 min, it is difficult to conclude that PSIS is inferior to SBS. Therefore, either SBS or PSIS placement can be selected according to each endoscopist's expertise or preference.

Our study has some limitations. The first is its retrospective design. The method of stent placement was not randomized. There is a difference in the background between the SBS group and the PSIS group. Although propensity score matching is useful to match the backgrounds of both groups, it was not performed in this study due to the small sample size. Second, various stents are used, and clinical outcomes may differ according to stent type. It would be ideal to compare SBS and PSIS using the same type of stent, but in practice, it is difficult to secure a sufficient sample size. Third, our study population, which comprised patients with different types of diseases, was heterogeneous. The time to stent occlusion may vary depending on the type of disease that causes UHMBS. To resolve this limitation, it is desirable to conduct the investigation for hilar cholangiocarcinoma only. However, it is still difficult to secure a sufficient sample size. Finally, the treatment of the second or third RBO has not been evaluated. Further analysis including long-term follow-up is necessary to mitigate this limitation.

5. Conclusions

PSIS has a significantly longer procedure time, despite the higher rate of expert enforcement in PSIS than in SBS. Moreover, the procedure of choice may be selected based on the endoscopist's experience and preference.

Author Contributions: Conceptualization, K.T. and H.O.; methodology, K.T. and H.O.; formal analysis, K.T.; investigation, M.K., M.O., H.N. and I.O.; data curation, M.K., M.O., H.N. and I.O.; writing—original draft preparation, K.T. and H.O.; writing—review and editing, all authors.; supervision, Y.T. and N.K; project administration, K.T., H.O., Y.T. and N.K.; All authors have read and agreed to the published version of the manuscript.

Funding: This study received no external funding.

Institutional Review Board Statement: The study was conducted in accordance with the Declaration of Helsinki, and approved by the Ethics Committee of Chiba University Hospital (protocol code: M10339 and date of approval: 6 February 2023).

Informed Consent Statement: Written informed consent for the procedure was obtained from all the patients. Consent for study participation was obtained using an opt-out methodology.

Data Availability Statement: The datasets generated during and/or analyzed during the current study are not publicly available but are available from the corresponding author upon reasonable request.

Conflicts of Interest: The authors declare no conflict of interest.

References

1. Pavlidis, E.T.; Pavlidis, T.E. Pathophysiological consequences of obstructive jaundice and perioperative management. *Hepatobiliary Pancreat. Dis. Int.* **2018**, *17*, 17–21. [CrossRef] [PubMed]
2. Wagner, H.J.; Knyrim, K.; Vakil, N.; Klose, K.J. Plastic endoprostheses versus metal stents in the palliative treatment of malignant hilar biliary obstruction. A prospective and randomized trial. *Endoscopy* **1993**, *25*, 213–218. [CrossRef] [PubMed]
3. Mukai, T.; Yasuda, I.; Nakashima, M.; Doi, S.; Iwashita, T.; Iwata, K.; Kato, T.; Tomita, E.; Moriwaki, H. Metallic stents are more efficacious than plastic stents in unresectable malignant hilar biliary strictures: A randomized controlled trial. *J. Hepatobiliary Pancreat. Sci.* **2013**, *20*, 214–222. [CrossRef]
4. Freeman, M.L.; Overby, C. Selective MRCP and CT-targeted drainage of malignant hilar biliary obstruction with self-expanding metallic stents. *Gastrointest. Endosc.* **2003**, *58*, 41–49. [CrossRef] [PubMed]
5. Vienne, A.; Hobeika, E.; Gouya, H.; Lapidus, N.; Fritsch, J.; Choury, A.D.; Chryssostalis, A.; Gaudric, M.; Pelletier, G.; Buffet, C.; et al. Prediction of drainage effectiveness during endoscopic stenting of malignant hilar strictures: The role of liver volume assessment. *Gastrointest. Endosc.* **2010**, *72*, 728–735. [CrossRef] [PubMed]
6. Takahashi, K.; Tsuyuguchi, T.; Saiga, A.; Horikoshi, T.; Ooka, Y.; Sugiyama, H.; Nakamura, M.; Kumagai, J.; Yamato, M.; Iino, Y.; et al. Risk factors of ineffective drainage in uncovered self-expandable metal stenting for unresectable malignant hilar biliary strictures. *Oncotarget* **2018**, *9*, 28185–28194. [CrossRef] [PubMed]
7. Lee, T.H.; Kim, T.H.; Moon, J.H.; Lee, S.H.; Choi, H.J.; Hwangbo, Y.; Hyun, J.J.; Choi, J.H.; Jeong, S.; Kim, J.H.; et al. Bilateral versus unilateral placement of metal stents for inoperable high-grade malignant hilar biliary strictures: A multicenter, prospective, randomized study (with video). *Gastrointest. Endosc.* **2017**, *86*, 817–827. [CrossRef] [PubMed]
8. Isayama, H.; Hamada, T.; Yasuda, I.; Itoi, T.; Ryozawa, S.; Nakai, Y.; Kogure, H.; Koike, K. TOKYO criteria 2014 for transpapillary biliary stenting. *Dig. Endosc.* **2015**, *27*, 259–264. [CrossRef]
9. De Palma, G.D.; Pezzullo, A.; Rega, M.; Persico, M.; Patrone, F.; Mastantuono, L.; Persico, G. Unilateral placement of metallic stents for malignant hilar obstruction: A prospective study. *Gastrointest. Endosc.* **2003**, *58*, 50–53. [CrossRef]
10. Kawamoto, H.; Tsutsumi, K.; Harada, R.; Fujii, M.; Kato, H.; Hirao, K.; Kurihara, N.; Nakanishi, T.; Mizuno, O.; Ishida, E.; et al. Endoscopic deployment of multiple JOSTENT SelfX is effective and safe in treatment of malignant hilar biliary strictures. *Clin. Gastroenterol. Hepatol.* **2008**, *6*, 401–408. [CrossRef]
11. Park, D.H.; Lee, S.S.; Moon, J.H.; Choi, H.J.; Cha, S.W.; Kim, J.H.; Seo, D.W.; Lee, S.K.; Park, S.H.; Lee, M.S.; et al. Newly designed stent for endoscopic bilateral stent-in-stent placement of metallic stents in patients with malignant hilar biliary strictures: Multicenter prospective feasibility study (with videos). *Gastrointest. Endosc.* **2009**, *69*, 1357–1360. [CrossRef] [PubMed]
12. Lee, J.H.; Kang, D.H.; Kim, J.Y.; Lee, S.M.; Kim, D.H.; Park, C.W.; Cho, H.S.; Kim, G.H.; Kim, T.O.; Heo, J.; et al. Endoscopic bilateral metal stent placement for advanced hilar cholangiocarcinoma: A pilot study of a newly designed Y stent. *Gastrointest. Endosc.* **2007**, *66*, 364–369. [CrossRef] [PubMed]
13. Kim, J.Y.; Kang, D.H.; Kim, H.W.; Choi, C.W.; Kim, I.D.; Hwang, J.H.; Kim, D.U.; Eum, J.S.; Bae, Y.M. Usefulness of slimmer and open-cell-design stents for endoscopic bilateral stenting and endoscopic revision in patients with hilar cholangiocarcinoma (with video). *Gastrointest. Endosc.* **2009**, *70*, 1109–1115. [CrossRef] [PubMed]
14. Chahal, P.; Baron, T.H. Expandable metal stents for endoscopic bilateral stent-within-stent placement for malignant hilar biliary obstruction. *Gastrointest. Endosc.* **2010**, *71*, 195–199. [CrossRef]
15. Naitoh, I.; Hayashi, K.; Nakazawa, T.; Okumura, F.; Miyabe, K.; Shimizu, S.; Yoshida, M.; Yamashita, H.; Ohara, H.; Joh, T. Side-by-side versus stent-in-stent deployment in bilateral endoscopic metal stenting for malignant hilar biliary obstruction. *Dig. Dis. Sci.* **2012**, *57*, 3279–3285. [CrossRef] [PubMed]
16. Kim, K.M.; Lee, K.H.; Chung, Y.H.; Shin, J.U.; Lee, J.K.; Lee, K.T.; Shim, S.G. A comparison of bilateral stenting methods for malignant hilar biliary obstruction. *Hepatogastroenterology* **2012**, *59*, 341–346. [CrossRef]
17. Lee, T.H.; Moon, J.H.; Choi, J.H.; Lee, S.H.; Lee, Y.N.; Paik, W.H.; Jang, D.K.; Cho, B.W.; Yang, J.K.; Hwangbo, Y.; et al. Prospective comparison of endoscopic bilateral stent-in-stent versus stent-by-stent deployment for inoperable advanced malignant hilar biliary stricture. *Gastrointest. Endosc.* **2019**, *90*, 222–230. [CrossRef]
18. Ishigaki, K.; Hamada, T.; Nakai, Y.; Isayama, H.; Sato, T.; Hakuta, R.; Saito, K.; Saito, T.; Takahara, N.; Mizuno, S.; et al. Retrospective Comparative Study of Side-by-Side and Stent-in-Stent Metal Stent Placement for Hilar Malignant Biliary Obstruction. *Dig. Dis. Sci.* **2020**, *65*, 3710–3718. [CrossRef]

19. Iwai, T.; Kida, M.; Okuwaki, K.; Yamauchi, H.; Kaneko, T.; Hasegawa, R.; Watanabe, M.; Kurosu, T.; Imaizumi, H.; Koizumi, W. Endoscopic re-intervention after stent-in-stent versus side-by-side bilateral self-expandable metallic stent deployment. *J. Gastroenterol. Hepatol.* **2022**, *37*, 1060–1066. [CrossRef]
20. Mehta, P.P.; Sanaka, M.R.; Parsi, M.A.; Albeldawi, M.J.; Dumot, J.A.; Lopez, R.; Zuccaro, G.; Vargo, J.J. Association of procedure length on outcomes and adverse events of endoscopic retrograde cholangiopancreatography. *Gastroenterol. Rep.* **2014**, *2*, 140–144. [CrossRef]
21. Kawanishi, K.; Kato, J.; Toda, N.; Yamagami, M.; Yamada, T.; Kojima, K.; Ohki, T.; Seki, M.; Tagawa, K. Risk Factors for Aspiration Pneumonia After Endoscopic Hemostasis. *Dig. Dis. Sci.* **2016**, *61*, 835–840. [CrossRef] [PubMed]
22. Park, K.; Kim, N.Y.; Kim, K.J.; Oh, C.; Chae, D.; Kim, S.Y. A Simple Risk Scoring System for Predicting the Occurrence of Aspiration Pneumonia After Gastric Endoscopic Submucosal Dissection. *Anesth. Analg.* **2022**, *134*, 114–122. [CrossRef] [PubMed]

Journal of *Personalized Medicine*

MDPI

Article

Clinical-Pathological Characteristics of Adenosquamous Esophageal Carcinoma: A Propensity-Score-Matching Study

Xinxin Xu [1,†], Feng Jiang [2,†], Yihan Guo [3], Hu Chen [1], Jiayi Qian [4], Leilei Wu [4], Dong Xie [4,*] and Guangxia Chen [5,*]

1 Department of Gastroenterology, The Affiliated Clinical College of Xuzhou Medical University, Xuzhou 221002, China
2 Department of Oncology, Zhongda Hospital, Southeast University, Nanjing 210009, China
3 Department of Scientific Research, Shaanxi Academy of Social Sciences, Xi'an 710061, China
4 Department of Thoracic Surgery, Shanghai Pulmonary Hospital, Tongji University, Shanghai 200092, China
5 Department of Gastroenterology, The Affiliated Xuzhou Municipal Hospital of Xuzhou Medical University, Xuzhou 221002, China
* Correspondence: xiedong@tongji.edu.cn (D.X.); gx_chen2010@163.com (G.C.)
† These authors contributed equally to this work.

Abstract: There are few studies on esophageal adenosquamous carcinoma (ADSC). Our study intended to investigate the clinical and survival features of ADSC. We included esophageal cancer (EC) data from the Surveillance, Epidemiology, and End Results program database to explore clinical and survival traits. Propensity score matching (PSM), the multivariate Cox regression model, and survival curves were used in this study. A total of 137 patients with ADSC were included in our analysis. The proportion of ADSC within the EC cohort declined from 2004 to 2018. Besides, results indicated no significant difference in survival between ADSC and SCC groups (PSM-adjusted HR = 1.249, $P = 0.127$). However, the survival rate of the ADSC group was significantly worse than that of the ADC group (PSM-adjusted HR = 1.497, $P = 0.007$). For the ADSC group, combined treatment with surgery had a higher survival rate than other treatment methods (all $P < 0.001$). Surgical resection, radiotherapy, and chemotherapy were independent protective prognostic factors (all $P < 0.05$). The proportion of ADSC has been declining from 2004 to 2018. The prognosis of ADSC is not significantly different from that of SCC but is worse than that of ADC. Surgery, radiotherapy, and chemotherapy could improve the prognosis of patients. Comprehensive treatment with surgery as the main treatment is more beneficial for some patients.

Keywords: esophageal adenosquamous carcinoma; propensity score matching; survival; proportion

1. Introduction

The latest global cancer statistics indicated that esophageal cancer (EC) is one of the most common primary gastrointestinal malignancies throughout the world [1]. It is reported that EC was the eighth-most common malignancy (new EC cases, N = 604,000) and the sixth-most common cause of cancer-related mortality (new EC deaths, N = 544,000) worldwide in 2020 [2]. Common pathologic types of EC contain esophageal squamous cell carcinoma (SCC) and adenocarcinoma (ADC). In addition, the incidence of EC varies geographically among different subtypes [3]. SCC incidence is highest in East Asia, while ADC incidence is highest in Northern Europe. Although SCC remains the most common type of EC worldwide, the incidence of ADC exceeds that of SCC in some high-income countries [4]. As early clinical symptoms of EC are not obvious, most patients are in the middle- and late-stage disease when they visit the hospital. The traditional treatments for EC are surgical resection, radiotherapy, chemotherapy, and molecular targeted therapy. In recent years, promising treatments for EC are emerging, but the prognosis of patients remains unsatisfactory and the 5-year overall survival (OS) rate still ranges from 15 to

25% [5]. Therefore, it is essential to evaluate the prognoses of EC and identify prognostic features in patients.

Primary adenosquamous carcinoma (ADSC), characterized by low incidence, high invasiveness, and poor prognosis, is an extremely rare histological type of EC [6]. Although the biological characteristic of ADSC is similar to that of ADC and SCC, it is not a simple fusion of these two types. There is no consensus in the current literature regarding the diagnostic criteria for ADSC in the digestive system. The 2010 edition of the *World Health Organization Classification of Gastrointestinal Neoplasms* did not define the proportion of ADC and SCC in the diagnosis for ADSC [7]. According to the criteria established by the Japanese Society of Esophagus, the diagnosis criteria of esophageal ADSC are two common histological types (ADC and SCC) accounting for more than 20% each [8]. This rare histological type accounts for about 0.9% of EC [9]. Because of the low incidence rate of ADSC, previous studies have mainly focused on ADC and SCC [10–12]. Currently, there are not many studies on the clinicopathological characteristics and survival analysis of ADSC in the world, so in this study, we decided to use the method of propensity score matching (PSM) to contrast the clinical characteristics and prognosis of ADSC and other two common tumor types from 2004 to 2018 using the Surveillance, Epidemiology, and End Results (SEER) program database, aiming to provide some reference value for clinicians' judgment on the improvement of the diagnosis and treatment levels and prognosis of ADSC.

2. Materials and Methods

2.1. Patient Selection

The SEER database is the cancer epidemiology and official source of cancer statistics. The SEER database includes cancer incidence and survival population data, relying on cancer registries in 19 geographic areas of the United States, covering morbidity, mortality, and prevalence information for approximately 35% of the US population [13]. Data on nine types of cancer cases are included in the SEER database, and cancer incidence is compared to the proportion of the population living. Through the analysis of these data, we can assimilate the cancer burden and its development trend and provide a basis for the formulation of prevention and control policies.

The Ethics Committee of Xuzhou Medical University Affiliated Municipal Hospital ratified the study, claiming that it dispensed with an ethical review because existing data on patient identity information were hidden. Informed consent was not required. We studied the patients in the SEER database who were definitively diagnosed with EC from 2004 to 2018. These patients were over 19 years old. In total, 44,948 patients with EC were involved after initial case selection. For further analysis of survival, our inclusion criteria were as follows: diagnosed as ADC, SCC, or ADSC tumors. We excluded patients who were diagnosed between 2016 and 2018, died within 1 month of diagnosis, or had less than 5 years of follow-up for inventory status. As SEER database information is currently only updated until 2020, cases from 2016 to 2018 were excluded because the 5-year survival rate was not available. The complete selection criteria are in Figure 1. Basic information gathered from the SEER database included sex, race/ethnicity, marital status, age at diagnosis, diagnosis year, and survival time. Tumor characteristics included the primary location (upper, middle, and lower thoracic esophagus), differentiation degree, TNM classification, histological subtype, and therapeutic method (e.g., surgery, radiotherapy, and chemotherapy). Overall survival (OS) and cancer-specific survival (CSS) were considered as the primary end points of this study.

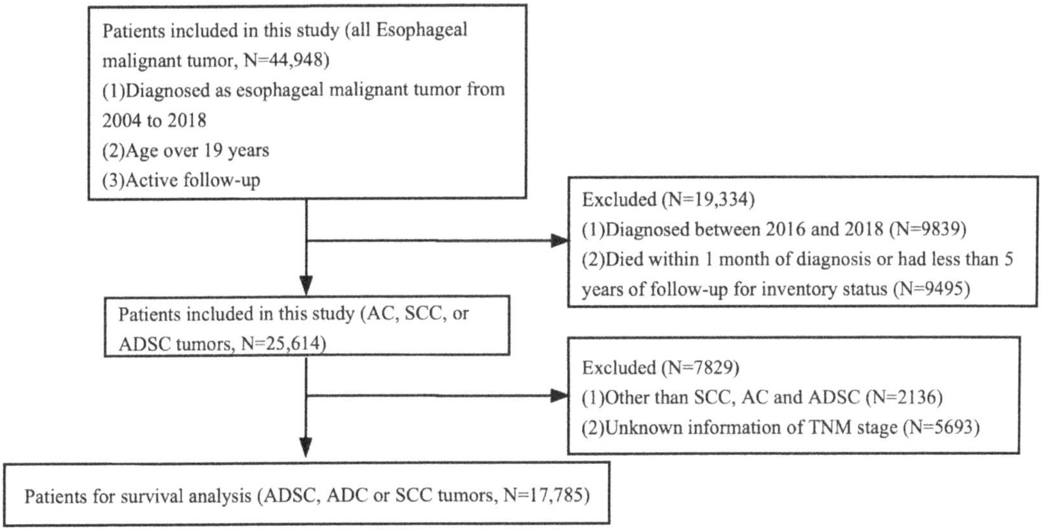

Figure 1. The flowchart of this study.

2.2. Propensity Score Matching

In this paper, gender, age, marital status, tumor site, TNM stage, and other pathological characteristics were used as matching variables. The propensity matching score was achieved using SPSS and SPSSAU, and the correction threshold was set as 0.1. The difference in baseline characteristics between the two groups was matched in a 1:1 ratio.

2.3. Statistical Analysis

All statistical analysis was performed using SPSS Statistics 25.0 software (IBM SPSS, Inc., Armonk, IL, USA) and GraphPad Prism 8 (Version 8.4.3). The chi-square test was performed to compare the differences in clinical baseline characteristics. The trend in the proportion of ADSC in the entire cohort was plotted. Risk ratios (RRs), and hazard ratios (HRs) and 95% confidence intervals (CIs) were calculated using multivariable logistic regression analysis and Cox regression analysis, respectively (the regression method was Enter selection). A multivariate Cox regression model was established, and survival curves were drawn to determine the survival in EC of different pathological types. Multivariable Cox regression analysis was conducted according to the results of the univariable analysis to determine independent prognosis factors. To prevent the statistical results from being affected by missing data, we also performed Cox regression analysis and plotted survival curves using the original data of 44,948 patients with EC to confirm the reliability of the results. Two-sided $P < 0.05$ was considered statistically significant.

3. Results

3.1. Patient Characteristics

Our study initially identified 44,948 cases diagnosed with EC from 2004 to 2018. After screening, we finally included 17,785 EC cases for survival analysis, including 137 ADSC cases, of which 100 patients with ADSC died in the cohort at the end of follow-up. The number of male patients with ADSC (N = 106) was more than that of females (N = 31), and the age distribution was homogenized in this cohort. We analyzed the anatomical location of ADSC, and the data showed that ADSC mainly occurred in the lower thoracic esophagus (N = 92, 67.2%), followed by the middle thoracic esophagus (N = 34, 24.8%). In accordance with the 8th edition of the *American Joint Committee on Cancer* staging system for SCC, 38 (27.7%) cases of cancers invaded the musculature propria, the musculature, or the submucosa (T1); 15 cases (10.9%) invaded the musculature propria (T2); 62 cases (45.3%) involved the tunica adventitia (T3); and 22 cases (16.1%) invaded local structures (T4). For the N stage, 81 (59.1%) patients had lymph node metastasis (N+). The detailed characteristic information about the patients is presented in Table 1. Finally, 17,785 patients met our selection criteria and were further analyzed using PSM. There were significant differences in sex, age, race, marital status, location, TNM stage, surgery, and grade before matching (Table 1). We adopted the PSM method to balance the differences in baseline characteristics between the groups. Finally, 411 patients were selected according to the ratio of 1:1, including 137 patients in the ADSC group, 137 patients in the SCC group, and 137 patients in the ADC group. A comparison of the baseline characteristics between the matched groups showed that the differences in baseline characteristics between the groups significantly reduced, as shown in Table 2.

Table 1. Baseline characteristics of three different pathological types of esophageal cancer in the SEER database (N (%)).

	ADSC (N = 137)	SCC (N = 6220)	ADC (N = 11,428)	χ^2	*P*-Value
Sex				1157.654	<0.001 [ab]
Female	31 (22.6%)	2177 (35.0%)	1509 (13.2%)		
Male	106 (77.4%)	4043 (65.0%)	9919 (86.8%)		
Age				6.816	0.033
<65 years	57 (41.6%)	2646 (42.5%)	5090 (44.5%)		
>64 years	80 (58.4%)	3574 (57.5%)	6338 (55.5%)		
Race				3493.035	<0.001 [ab]
White patients	119 (86.9%)	3692 (59.4%)	10,838 (94.8%)		
Other patients	18 (13.1%)	2528 (40.6%)	590 (5.2%)		
Marital status				543.109	<0.001 [b]
Unmarried	62 (45.3%)	3150 (50.6%)	3805 (33.3%)		
Married	72 (52.6%)	2795 (44.9%)	7154 (62.6%)		
Unknown	3 (2.2%)	275 (4.4%)	469 (4.1%)		
Location				6441.786	<0.001 [ab]
Upper thoracic esophagus	4 (2.9%)	1002 (16.1%)	117 (1.0%)		
Middle thoracic esophagus	34 (24.8%)	2634 (42.3%)	733 (6.4%)		
Lower thoracic esophagus	92 (67.2%)	2060 (33.1%)	10,342 (90.5%)		
Unknown	7 (5.1%)	524 (8.4%)	236 (2.1%)		
Radiotherapy				149.737	<0.001
No	41 (29.9%)	1742 (28.0%)	4239 (37.1%)		
Yes	95 (69.3%)	4415 (71.0%)	7095 (62.1%)		
Unknown	1 (0.7%)	63 (1.0%)	94 (0.8%)		
Chemotherapy				5.637	0.060
No	42 (30.7%)	2056 (33.1%)	3580 (31.3%)		
Yes	95 (69.3%)	4164 (66.9%)	7848 (68.7%)		
Surgery				771.160	<0.001 [a]
None	89 (65.0%)	4887 (78.6%)	6637 (58.1%)		
Local treatment	1 (0.7%)	109 (1.8%)	607 (5.3%)		
Surgical resection	46 (33.6%)	1190 (19.1%)	4089 (35.8%)		
Unknown	1 (0.7%)	34 (0.5%)	95 (0.8%)		
Grade				164.213	<0.001 [ab]
I	0 (0.0%)	318 (5.1%)	610 (5.3%)		
II	20 (14.6%)	2627 (42.2%)	4031 (35.3%)		
III–IV	96 (70.1%)	2210 (35.5%)	4906 (42.9%)		
Unknown	21 (15.3%)	1065 (17.1%)	1881 (16.5%)		
T				109.641	<0.001
T1	38 (27.7%)	2087 (33.6%)	3955 (34.6%)		
T2	15 (10.9%)	780 (12.5%)	1471 (12.9%)		
T3	62 (45.3%)	2270 (36.5%)	4638 (40.6%)		
T4	22 (16.1%)	1083 (17.4%)	1364 (11.9%)		

Table 1. *Cont.*

	ADSC (N = 137)	SCC (N = 6220)	ADC (N = 11,428)	χ^2	*P*-Value
N				18.875	0.016
N0	56 (40.9%)	3023 (48.6%)	5258 (46.0%)		
N+	81 (59.1%)	3197 (51.4%)	6170 (54.0%)		
M				71.458	<0.001
M0	98 (71.5%)	5048 (81.2%)	8653 (75.7%)		
M1	39 (28.5%)	1172 (18.8%)	2775 (24.3%)		

Note: Compared with the SCC group, ADSC group [a] $P < 0.05$; compared with the ADC group, ADSC group [b] $P < 0.05$.

Table 2. Demographic and clinical characteristics of the three groups after PSM (N (%)).

	ADSC (N = 137)	SCC (N = 137)	ADC (N = 137)	χ^2	*P*
Sex				2.450	0.294
Female	31 (22.6%)	33 (24.1%)	23 (16.8%)		
Male	106 (77.4%)	104 (75.9%)	114 (83.2%)		
Age				2.187	0.335
<65 years	57 (41.6%)	68 (49.6%)	58 (42.3%)		
>64 years	80 (58.4%)	69 (50.4%)	79 (57.7%)		
Surgery				4.541	0.604
None	89 (65%)	94 (68.6%)	85 (62%)		
Local treatment	1 (0.7%)	1 (0.7%)	0 (0%)		
Surgical resection	46 (33.6%)	42 (30.7%)	52 (38%)		
Unknown	1 (0.7%)	0 (0%)	0 (0%)		
Radiotherapy				4.036	0.401
No	41 (29.9%)	32 (23.4%)	41 (29.9%)		
Yes	95 (69.3%)	105 (76.6%)	96 (70.1%)		
Unknown	1 (0.7%)	0 (0%)	0 (0%)		
Chemotherapy				3.602	0.165
No	42 (30.7%)	32 (23.4%)	29 (21.2%)		
Yes	95 (69.3%)	105 (76.6%)	108 (78.8%)		
Marital status				5.799	0.215
Unmarried	62 (45.3%)	64 (46.7%)	52 (38%)		
Married	72 (52.6%)	71 (51.8%)	85 (62%)		
Unknown	3 (2.2%)	2 (1.5%)	0 (0%)		
Grade				10.387	0.109
I	0 (0%)	0 (0%)	4 (2.9%)		
II	20 (14.6%)	28 (20.4%)	28 (20.4%)		
III IV	96 (70.1%)	90 (65.7%)	87 (63.5%)		
Unknown	21 (15.3%)	19 (13.9%)	18 (13.1%)		
Location				23.427	0.001 [b]
Upper thoracic esophagus	4 (2.9%)	8 (5.8%)	1 (0.7%)		
Middle thoracic esophagus	34 (24.8%)	39 (28.5%)	17 (12.4%)		
Lower thoracic esophagus	92 (67.2%)	84 (61.3%)	117 (85.4%)		
unknown	7 (5.1%)	6 (4.4%)	2 (1.5%)		
T				6.892	0.331
T1	38 (27.7%)	46 (33.6%)	41 (29.9%)		
T2	15 (10.9%)	16 (11.7%)	10 (7.3%)		
T3	62 (45.3%)	54 (39.4%)	72 (52.6%)		
T4	22 (16.1%)	21 (15.3%)	14 (10.2%)		
N				3.683	0.451
N0	56 (40.9%)	59 (43.1%)	60 (43.8%)		
N1	3 (2.2%)	0 (0%)	1 (0.7%)		
N2	0 (0%)	0 (0%)	0 (0%)		
N3	78 (56.9%)	78 (56.9%)	76 (55.5%)		
N+	0 (0%)	0 (0%)	0 (0%)		

Table 2. *Cont.*

	ADSC (N = 137)	SCC (N = 137)	ADC (N = 137)	χ^2	*P*
M				3.992	0.136
M0	98 (71.5%)	110 (80.3%)	97 (70.8%)		
M1	39 (28.5%)	27 (19.7%)	40 (29.2%)		

Note: Compared with the ADC group, ADSC group [b] $P < 0.05$.

3.2. Proportion of ADSC

The proportion of ADSC in the entire cohort was 0.7 per 100 patients and decreased from 2004 to 2018 (Figure 2; 0.834 per 100 patients (95% CI 0.005–0.012) in 2004; 0.548 per 100 patients (95% CI 0.003–0.008) in 2018). Among the 44,948 cases in the EC cohort, the largest proportion of ADC showed a continuous increase year by year, with a slow decrease in the proportion of SCC (Figure 3). Multivariable logistic regression indicated that the proportion of ADSC presented a declined trend over the year (Table 3; adjusted RR = 0.972, 95% CI 0.947–0.998, $P = 0.037$). In addition, linear regression analysis led to the same results ($R = 0.578$, $P < 0.05$). In addition, the high incidence rate among Caucasians was significant (adjusted RR = 1.461, 95% CI 1.045–2.044, $P = 0.027$).

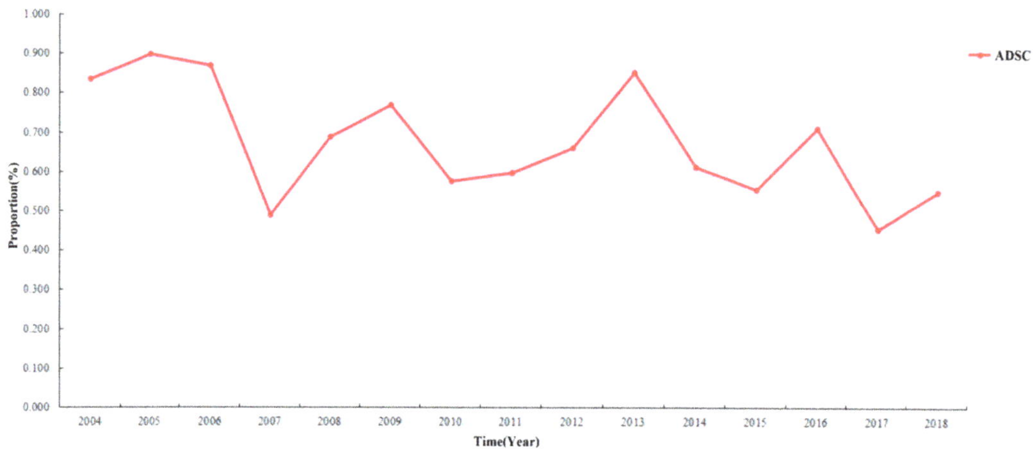

Time(Year)	2004	2005	2006	2007	2008	2009	2010	2011	2012	2013	2014	2015	2016	2017	2018
ADSC	23	23	23	14	20	23	17	18	20	26	19	18	23	15	18
All cancers	2758	2560	2650	2854	2905	2992	2952	3017	3021	3054	3100	3246	3243	3312	3284
Proportion(%)	0.834	0.898	0.868	0.491	0.688	0.769	0.576	0.597	0.662	0.851	0.613	0.555	0.709	0.453	0.548
95%CI	0.005–0.012	0.005–0.013	0.005–0.012	0.002–0.007	0.004–0.01	0.005–0.011	0.003–0.008	0.003–0.009	0.004–0.01	0.005–0.012	0.003–0.009	0.003–0.008	0.004–0.01	0.002–0.007	0.003–0.008

Figure 2. The proportion of esophageal adenosquamous carcinoma over time in the 44,948 patients with esophageal cancer.

Table 3. The results of multivariable logistic regression analyses.

	Multivariable Analysis		
	RR	95% CI	*P*-Value
Sex (male = 1 vs. female = 0)	1.115	0.838–1.484	0.455
Year of diagnosis (continuous)	0.972	0.947–0.998	0.037
Age (<65 years = 0 vs. ≥65 years = 1)	0.910	0.722–1.147	0.424
Race (Caucasians = 1 vs. others = 0)	1.461	1.045–2.044	0.027

Note: The results of multivariable analysis were adjusted for other confounding factors, such as sex, age, and race/ethnicity. RR: risk ratio; CI: confidence interval. The logistic regression method was Enter selection.

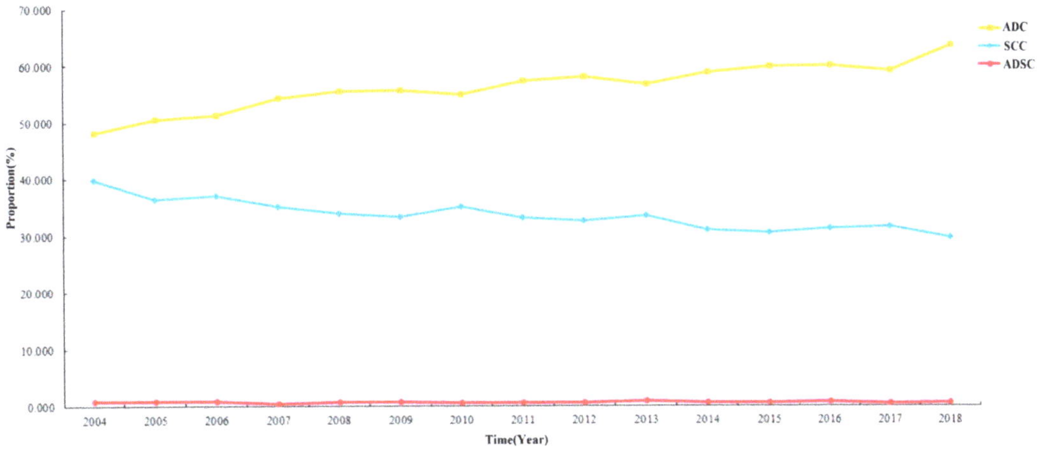

Time(Year)	2004	2005	2006	2007	2008	2009	2010	2011	2012	2013	2014	2015	2016	2017	2018
ADC	1331	1296	1361	1548	1613	1665	1620	1726	1753	1729	1819	1941	1944	1955	2085
All cancers	2758	2560	2650	2854	2905	2992	2952	3017	3021	3054	3100	3246	3243	3312	3284
Proportion(%)	48.260	50.625	51.358	54.240	55.525	55.648	54.878	57.209	58.027	56.614	58.677	59.797	59.944	59.028	63.490
95%CI	0.464–0.501	0.487–0.526	0.495–0.533	0.524–0.561	0.537–0.573	0.539–0.574	0.531–0.567	0.554–0.59	0.563–0.598	0.549–0.584	0.569–0.604	0.581–0.615	0.583–0.616	0.574–0.607	0.618–0.651
SCC	1099	934	982	1004	987	997	1036	1002	984	1023	959	992	1014	1045	975
All cancers	2758	2560	2650	2854	2905	2992	2952	3017	3021	3054	3100	3246	3243	3312	3284
Proportion(%)	39.848	36.484	37.057	35.179	33.976	33.322	35.095	33.212	32.572	33.497	30.935	30.561	31.267	31.552	29.689
95%CI	0.38–0.417	0.346–0.384	0.352–0.389	0.334–0.369	0.323–0.357	0.316–0.35	0.334–0.368	0.315–0.349	0.309–0.342	0.318–0.352	0.293–0.326	0.29–0.321	0.297–0.329	0.3–0.331	0.281–0.313
ADSC	23	23	23	14	20	23	17	18	20	26	19	18	23	15	18
All cancers	2758	2560	2650	2854	2905	2992	2952	3017	3021	3054	3100	3246	3243	3312	3284
Proportion(%)	0.834	0.898	0.868	0.491	0.688	0.769	0.576	0.597	0.662	0.851	0.613	0.555	0.709	0.453	0.548
95%CI	0.005–0.012	0.005–0.013	0.005–0.012	0.002–0.007	0.004–0.01	0.005–0.011	0.003–0.008	0.003–0.009	0.004–0.01	0.005–0.012	0.003–0.009	0.003–0.008	0.004–0.01	0.002–0.007	0.003–0.008

Figure 3. The crude incidence rate of three different pathological types of esophageal cancer over time in 44,948 patients.

3.3. Survival Analysis of Histology Classification

Our results showed that the survival rate of EC was at a low level. We found no significant difference in survival between the ADSC group and the more common histological classification of EC in the results of the multivariable analysis before PSM. Patients with SCC (unadjusted HR = 1.081, $P < 0.05$) had a worse prognosis than patients with ADC. The unadjusted survival curves were consistent with these results (Figure 4A). After PSM, data analysis showed that the median survival time of ADC, SCC, and ADSC was 15 months (95% CI 11.0–20.0 months), 12 months (95% CI 10.0–15.0 months), and 11 months (5% CI 9.0–13.0 months), respectively. Besides, further analysis found that the survival rate of patients with ADSC (PSM-adjusted HR = 1.497, $P = 0.007$) was lower than that of patients with ADC (Figure 4B). We found that the SCC group had a higher survival rate than the ADSC group, but the difference was not statistically significant (PSM-adjusted HR = 1.249, $P = 0.127$; Figure 4C). The PSM-adjusted survival curve was consistent with these results. We performed survival analysis again using the pre-deletion data and obtained results that were generally consistent with our selection of patients by condition (see Supplementary Figure S1).

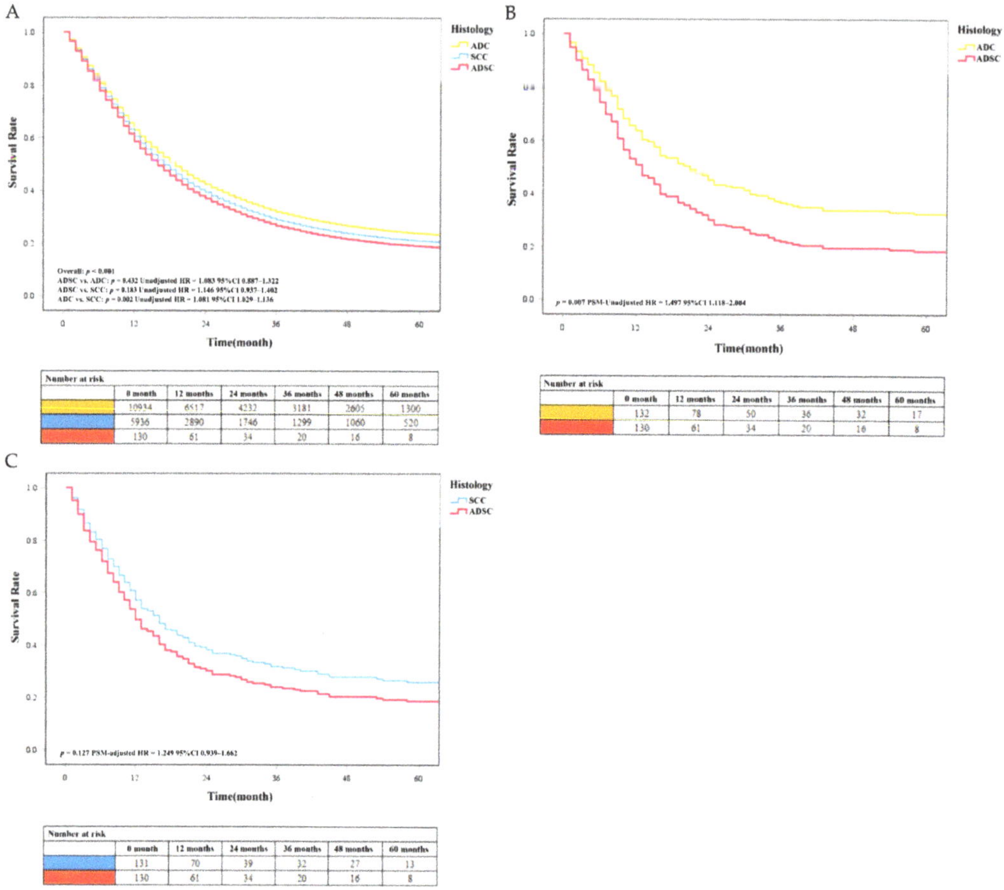

Figure 4. (**A**) The unadjusted survival curves of different histology classifications before PSM. The COX survival curves of EC with different histology classifications after PSM. (**B**) Survival comparison between the ADC and ADSC groups. (**C**) Survival comparison between the SCC and ADSC groups.

3.4. Survival Analysis of Different Treatment Groups in ADSC

According to the different treatment methods, patients with ADSC were divided into four groups: patients without surgery, radiotherapy, and chemotherapy were categorized into the untreated group (N = 9), patients who only underwent surgery without radiotherapy or chemotherapy were categorized into the surgery-only group (N = 15), patients without surgery but radiotherapy or chemotherapy were categorized into the chemoradiotherapy group (N = 79), and patients who underwent surgery, radiotherapy, and chemotherapy were categorized into the combined treatment group (N = 33). Survival analysis was performed on these four groups of patients (Figure 5). Cox survival curve analysis showed that the survival rate of patients in the combined treatment group was significantly higher than that in the other three groups ($P < 0.001$). The survival rate of patients in the surgery-only group was higher than that in chemoradiotherapy group. These results further confirmed that surgery combined with chemoradiotherapy has a higher clinical application value than chemoradiotherapy alone in patients with ADSC.

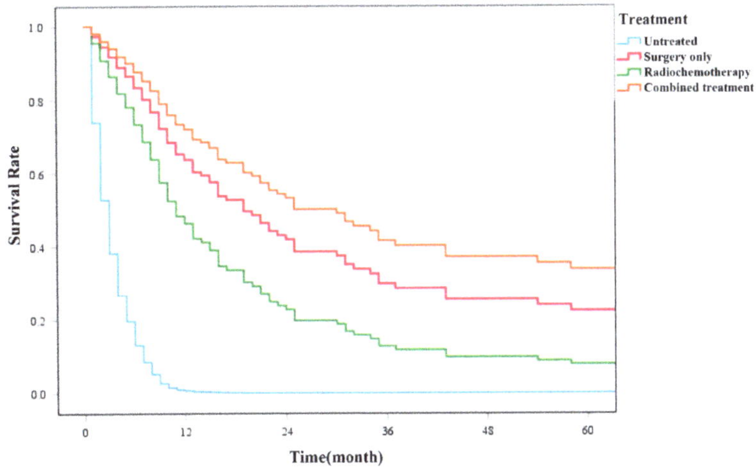

Number at risk						
	0 month	12 months	24 months	36 months	48 months	60 months
	9	0	0	0	0	0
	14	9	5	2	2	1
	74	30	12	7	5	3
	33	22	18	11	9	4

Figure 5. COX survival curves for different treatment groups of patients with ADSC.

3.5. Prognostic Analysis for ADSC

About one-third of the 137 patients with ADSC underwent surgery. The number of patients who received radiation therapy was 95 (69.3%), the same as those who received chemotherapy. The relationship between clinicopathological features and prognosis is presented in Table 4. Among them, surgical resection, radiotherapy, and chemotherapy could significantly improve the outcomes of patients (adjusted HR = 0.326, 95% CI 0.168–0.631, $P = 0.001$; adjusted HR = 0.532, 95% CI 0.299–0.949, $P = 0.032$; and adjusted HR = 0.409, 95% CI 0.215–0.777, $P = 0.006$, respectively). By adjusting for confounders, we identified surgical resection, radiotherapy, and chemotherapy as independent prognostic factors (Table 4). In addition, there were no significant differences in mortality by patients' sex, age, marital status, tumor differentiation, location of the tumor, and TNM classification in both univariable and multivariable analyses (all $P > 0.05$). The results of the Cox survival analysis of the 380 patients with ADSC before censoring were consistent with those after screening (see Supplementary Table S1).

Table 4. Univariable and multivariable Cox proportional hazard regression analyses for mortality in 137 patients with ADSC.

Variables	Univariable Analysis			Multivariable Analysis		
	HR	95% CI	*P*	HR	95% CI	*P*
Sex						
Female	1	Reference		1	Reference	
Male	0.952	0.600–1.509	0.833	1.010	0.595–1.717	0.969
Age						
<65 years	1	Reference		1	Reference	
>64 years	0.951	0.641–1.409	0.801	0.742	0.477–1.153	0.184
Surgery						
None	1	Reference		1	Reference	
Local treatment	1.428	0.197–10.361	0.725	3.930	0.352–43.871	0.266

Table 4. *Cont.*

Variables	Univariable Analysis			Multivariable Analysis		
	HR	95% CI	P	HR	95% CI	P
Surgical resection	0.419	0.269–0.653	0	0.326	0.168–0.631	0.001
Unknown	0.596	0.082–4.315	0.608	0.127	0.006–2.738	0.188
Radiotherapy						
No	1	Reference		1	Reference	
Yes	0.656	0.430–1.002	0.051	0.532	0.299–0.949	0.032
Unknown	7.593	0.977–59.007	0.053	3.703	0.407–33.716	0.245
Chemotherapy						
No	1	Reference		1	Reference	
Yes	0.627	0.408-0.965	0.034	0.409	0.215-0.777	0.006
Marital status						
Unmarried	1	Reference		1	Reference	
Married	0.709	0.476–1.057	0.092	1.016	0.618–1.672	0.949
Unknown	1.228	0.296–5.086	0.777	4.436	0.492–39.950	0.184
Grade						
II	1	Reference		1	Reference	
III–IV	1.070	0.602–1.903	0.818	0.994	0.515–1.918	0.986
Unknown	1.510	0.732–3.111	0.264	1.172	0.520–2.643	0.701
Location						
Upper thoracic esophagus	1	Reference		1	Reference	
Middle thoracic esophagus	0.523	0.181–1.509	0.231	0.928	0.234–3.683	0.915
Lower thoracic esophagus	0.490	0.178–1.353	0.169	1.023	0.262–3.993	0.974
Unknown	0.556	0.156–1.985	0.366	0.920	0.176–4.805	0.921
T						
T1	1	Reference		1	Reference	
T2	0.997	0.492–2.020	0.993	1.793	0.798–4.029	0.158
T3	0.674	0.416–1.092	0.109	1.048	0.598–1.835	0.871
T4	1.488	0.817–2.708	0.193	1.474	0.716–3.034	0.292
N						
N0	1	Reference		1	Reference	
N1	3.560	1.073–11.810	0.038	1.119	0.206–6.079	0.896
M						
M0	1	Reference		1	Reference	
M1	2.106	1.374–3.228	0.001	1.372	0.776–2.425	0.277

4. Discussion

ADSC is a relatively rare tumor. Besides, there is a lack of research to inform treatment recommendations and prognostic assessments for patients with ADSC. We used a large database to investigate the clinicopathological characteristics and prognostic factors of patients with ADSC. In addition, the patient outcomes for different treatment modalities are of great interest to clinicians in developing treatment plans and assessing prognosis. In this study, we used the data of 44,948 patients with EC to calculate the proportion of ADSC cases. The proportion of ADSC was 0.7% in our study, and the proportion of ADSC was on the decline between 2004 and 2018. Besides, 137 patients with ADSC were included in baseline characteristics analysis and further Cox regression analyses. According to the results, the survival rates in ADSC were similar to those in SCC but significantly lower than those in ADC. Gender, age, grade, and marital status were not independent protective prognostic factors for ADSC. By adjusting for confounders, surgical resection, radiotherapy, and chemotherapy were identified as independent prognostic factors. In addition, combined treatment with surgery was more effective than other treatment options in improving the survival rate. Therefore, we believe that comprehensive treatment based on surgical resection is the optimal treatment for some patients with ADSC.

The prognosis of esophageal malignant tumors is poor. Because their symptoms are hidden, most patients are already in the middle and late stages of clinical treatment. In this study, the disease of most patients was in the medium or low differentiation level, and more than half of them had metastasis of the lymph nodes. For patients with this disease staging, surgical treatment is often not recommended, which leads to the 5-year survival rate of the patients being less than 20% [14]. At present, ESCC mainly occurs in two-thirds of the stratified squamous epithelium of the esophagus. Histopathology can observe squamous differentiation of the esophageal epithelium; damage to basal and underlying structures; and matrix reactions, vascular lymphatic vessels, and peripheral nerves [15]. EC is common in men. A previous study found that sex hormone levels may be a factor affecting the gender difference in EC incidence [16]. In addition, EC is directly related to alcohol and tobacco consumption. Long-term tobacco and alcohol stimulation changes the tissue microenvironment, which can greatly increase the risk of cloning and evolution of cancer cells [17]. ADC usually occurs in the lower third of the esophageal mucosa, mainly originating from the Barrett mucosa. Since the 1970s, the incidence of ADC in Europe and the United States has gradually increased. One of the reasons may be the increase in the proportion of people with obesity, which increases the prevalence of gastroesophageal reflux. The lower esophageal mucosa is in a low-pH environment for a long time, and the risk of ADC also increases [2]. ADSC is more invasive than epidermal cancer, with a spread of more than 75% in local lymph nodes, distant metastasis of more than 25%, and a 5-year survival rate of 15–25% [15]. In fact, regardless of histology, the prognosis level of esophageal cancer is unsatisfactory. Only about 20% of patients can survive for 3 years or more after diagnosis [18]. Therefore, primary prevention and early diagnosis of EC require successful strategies. Primary prevention of EC mainly involves lifestyle changes, such as avoiding smoking and drinking alcohol; secondary preventions, such as endoscopy monitoring programs and chemical prophylaxis, are equally important.

ADSC is a special mixed cell type of EC and a comparatively scarce pathological type of EC, which means that the cancer tissue incorporates both SCC and ADC components. Due to the extremely low incidence of ADSC, most of the current studies on ADSC are isolated case reports or clinicopathological series reports [19–22]. However, the specific incidence and prognostic characteristics of ADSC in different countries or regions are not well described. According to the current literature, the proportion of ADSC is between 0.37 and 1% [23]. This study showed that the number of ADSC cases account for about 0.7% (300/44,948) of primary EC, which is basically consistent with literature reports. Furthermore, the proportion of ADSC in the entire EC alignment decreased from 2004 to 2018. The promotion of computed tomography and upper gastrointestinal endoscopy may have contributed to the decline in the overall trend [24–27].

However, the accuracy of upper gastrointestinal endoscopic biopsy in diagnosing ADSC is low. Preoperative endoscopic biopsy just diagnosed 1 (4.2%) case of ADSC in the study by Sun et al. [28]. Most patients were diagnosed with SCC on preoperative biopsy [20,29]. This might be because the SCC component was located in the mucosa, while the ADC component was mainly located in the deeper region of the tumor or in metastatic lymph nodes [23]. Another important reason was that almost all ADSCs were covered by normal epithelial cells or intraepithelial neoplasia [30]. A combination of magnifying endoscopy with narrow-band imaging (ME-NBI), endoscopic ultrasonography (EUS), and deeper biopsy potentially improves preoperative diagnostic accuracy [31].

At present, due to a lack of cases, there is no large sample of prospective randomized control results to clarify the biological characteristics and prognosis of ADSC, and there is also disagreement about the survival and prognosis in ADSC. Existing studies are controversial in comparing the prognosis in ADSC, ADC, and SCC. ADSC has been proven to be more aggressive than ADC and SCC alone, with a high rate of lymph node metastasis and inferior prognosis [21,32]. Most of the previous studies have found that the OS of patient with ADSC is worse than that of patient with ADC or SCC [19,33]. Data from Evans et al. showed that the 2- and 5-year OS rates in ADSC are 23.8 and 12.8%, respectively, which is lower in ADC and SCC [9]. Our results showed that ADSC survival is similar to SCC survival but inferior to ADC survival. We hypothesized that although ADSC confuses two different tumor components, the prognosis is not a general combination of the two.

Coincidentally, Yendamuri et al. and Chen et al. reported that the prognosis of ADSC is consistent with that of SCC [34,35]. In addition, Yachida et al. found that ADSC had better prognosis than SCC in their series of 18 patients with this disease [36]. This paradoxical result might be explained by the fact that the ADSC tumors included were early tumors with a low T status. Another possibility is that due to the small number of ADSC cases, there was selection bias of clinical factors, and sample size analysis needs to be further expanded to improve the accuracy.

Surgery, radiotherapy, and chemotherapy are the main treatment approaches for patients with EC [37,38], which were recognized as independent protective predictors of prognosis in our results. The prognosis of patients undergoing surgery and chemotherapy were better in both single-factor analysis and multi-factor analysis. Patients undergoing surgical resection have a superior prognosis, which is related to the clinical stage of ADSC, and in general, patients who get an opportunity for surgery tend to have earlier stages of the disease. In this study, 137 patients with ADSC were analyzed, and it was found that the prognosis was correlated with the selection of treatment methods and the difference was statistically significant. The survival time of patients treated with surgery combined with radiotherapy or chemotherapy was generally longer than that of patients treated with surgery alone. This may be because ADSC easily invades the surrounding tissues and organs, so surgical resection alone often cannot completely remove the cancer foci. Preoperative or postoperative chemoradiotherapy may help to remove the residual lesions, thus improving the survival time of patients. Therefore, it is believed that the preferred treatment of ADSC should be surgery assisted with local radiotherapy or chemotherapy, which is also a relatively recognized treatment method at present [39–41]. It is important to note that the cloning dynamics of cancer are altered by the introduction of drugs or radiation therapy, with consequent mass cell death, providing selective pressure on the proliferation of mutated cells. However, many chemotherapy drugs are genotoxic, and surviving cancer cells may develop genetic mutations that increase their fitness and malignancy potential. In addition, in recent years, drugs targeting the immune checkpoint mechanism are a new and widely used and effective means [42,43]. A large number of studies have shown that immunotherapy is effective for EC, a tumor with a high mutation burden, and has now become another effective treatment method for middle and advanced esophageal malignancies after surgical resection, radiotherapy, and chemotherapy.

Recent studies have reported that lymph node metastasis is the exclusive independent prognostic factor for ADSC [29,44]. In 2016, Qian et al. believed that after correcting the interference of other mixed factors, a higher combined stage, a frequent lymph node metastasis rate, and higher distant metastasis are associated with poor prognosis of ADSC [33]. Contrary to the findings of this previous study, our series did not find the tumor location, TNM stage of the tumor, and tumor grade affecting the prognosis of ADSC. The reason may be that some data were limited by the availability of the database. On average, 5.1% of cancers were classified as overlapping or unspecified locations and 15.3% of the patients were not clearly graded. Another reason is that the sample size included was relatively small, and the baseline level of included cases was uneven.

Our research still leaves something to be desired. First, we could not obtain some crucial information, such as distant metastases, the serous membrane invasion area, and the tumor infiltration depth, because we could not obtain exhaustive data of esophagoscopy and computerized tomography examination from the SEER database. Therefore, we did not conduct an in-depth classification and evaluation of ADSC. Second, this study lacked specific diagnosis and treatment information. We only compared the prognosis after surgical resection, radiotherapy, and chemotherapy, and the exact combination and sequence of treatments are unclear. Finally, since this study was retrospective, expanding the sample size analysis is required to further explore and verify the incidence, clinicopathological features, diagnosis, and prognostic factors of patients with ADSC.

5. Conclusions

ADSC is a special type of tumor different from SCC and ADC, and its prognosis is similar to that in SCC but significantly lower than that in ADC. Surgery, radiotherapy, and chemotherapy can improve the prognosis of patients. Comprehensive treatment with surgery as the main treatment is more beneficial for some patients. Further large-scale or multi-center randomized prospective trials are required to explore the biological behavior of esophageal ADSC, improve the accuracy of early diagnosis, and set more effective diagnostic guidelines and therapeutic strategies.

Supplementary Materials: The following supporting information can be downloaded at: https://www.mdpi.com/article/10.3390/jpm13030468/s1, Figure S1: curves of EC with three different histological classifications in the raw data. Table S1. Univariable and multivariable Cox proportion hazard regression analyses for mortality in 380 ADSC patients.

Author Contributions: Conceptualization, X.X., D.X., F.J. and G.C.; data curation, H.C. and L.W.; formal analysis, Y.G.; funding acquisition, G.C.; investigation, F.J.; methodology, Y.G.; software, H.C. and J.Q.; supervision, D.X.; validation, L.W.; visualization, J.Q.; writing—original draft, X.X.; writing—review and editing, G.C. All authors have read and agreed to the published version of the manuscript.

Funding: This research was funded by the "Xuzhou Municipal Health and Health Commission Medical Leading Talents Training Program" (grant number XWRCHT20210) and the "Xuzhou Science and Technology Plan Project" (grant number KC21169).

Institutional Review Board Statement: This study was approved by the Ethics Committee of the Xuzhou Medical University Affiliated Municipal Hospital. The SEER database is publicly available and provides de-identified case data. Because the analysis used pseudonymous clinical data, the subjects' written informed consent was waived. We confirm that all methods were performed in accordance with relevant guidelines and regulations.

Informed Consent Statement: Not applicable.

Data Availability Statement: The data sets generated and analyzed were obtained in the SEER database in April 2022 (https://seer.cancer.gov/). These data sets are available from the corresponding author upon reasonable request.

Acknowledgments: We thank the staff of the SEER program.

Conflicts of Interest: The authors declare no conflict of interest.

References

1. Dyba, T.; Randi, G.; Bray, F.; Martos, C.; Giusti, F.; Nicholson, N.; Gavin, A.; Flego, M.; Neamtiu, L.; Dimitrova, N.; et al. The European cancer burden in 2020: Incidence and mortality estimates for 40 countries and 25 major cancers. *Eur. J. Cancer* **2021**, *157*, 308–347. [CrossRef] [PubMed]
2. Arnold, M.; Ferlay, J.; van Berge Henegouwen, M.I.; Soerjomataram, I. Global burden of oesophageal and gastric cancer by histology and subsite in 2018. *Gut* **2020**, *69*, 1564–1571. [CrossRef]
3. Arnold, M.; Laversanne, M.; Brown, L.M.; Devesa, S.S.; Bray, F. Predicting the Future Burden of Esophageal Cancer by Histological Subtype: International Trends in Incidence up to 2030. *Am. J. Gastroenterol.* **2017**, *112*, 1247–1255. [CrossRef] [PubMed]
4. Pennathur, A.; Gibson, M.K.; Jobe, B.A.; Luketich, J.D. Oesophageal carcinoma. *Lancet* **2013**, *381*, 400–412. [CrossRef]
5. Sung, H.; Ferlay, J.; Siegel, R.L.; Laversanne, M.; Soerjomataram, I.; Jemal, A.; Bray, F. Global Cancer Statistics 2020: GLOBOCAN Estimates of Incidence and Mortality Worldwide for 36 Cancers in 185 Countries. *CA Cancer J. Clin.* **2021**, *71*, 209–249. [CrossRef] [PubMed]
6. Li, H.S.; He, T.; Yang, L. Adenosquamous carcinoma of the digestive system: A literature review. *Scand. J. Gastroenterol.* **2020**, *55*, 1268–1276. [CrossRef]
7. Fléjou, J.F. WHO Classification of digestive tumors: The fourth edition. *Ann. Pathol.* **2011**, *31* (Suppl. S5), S27-31. [CrossRef]
8. Japan Esophageal Society. Japanese Classification of Esophageal Cancer, 11th Edition: Part II and III. *Esophagus* **2017**, *14*, 37–65. [CrossRef]
9. Evans, M.; Liu, Y.; Chen, C.; Steuer, C.; Iii, R.C.; Landry, J.; Higgins, K.; Beitler, J.J.; Willingham, F.; Owonikoko, T.K.; et al. Adenosquamous Carcinoma of the Esophagus: An NCDB-Based Investigation on Comparative Features and Overall Survival in a Rare Tumor. *Oncology* **2017**, *93*, 336–342. [CrossRef]

10. Wu, L.-L.; Zhong, J.-D.; Zhu, J.-L.; Kang, L.; Huang, Y.-Y.; Lin, P.; Long, H.; Zhang, L.-J.; Ma, Q.-L.; Qiu, L.-H.; et al. Postoperative survival effect of the number of examined lymph nodes on esophageal squamous cell carcinoma with pathological stage T1–3N0M0. *BMC Cancer* **2022**, *22*, 1–11. [CrossRef]
11. Wu, L.-L.; Wang, J.-L.; Huang, W.; Liu, X.; Huang, Y.-Y.; Zeng, J.; Cui, C.-Y.; Lu, J.-B.; Lin, P.; Long, H.; et al. Prognostic Modeling of Patients Undergoing Surgery Alone for Esophageal Squamous Cell Carcinoma: A Histopathological and Computed Tomography Based Quantitative Analysis. *Front. Oncol.* **2021**, *11*, 565755. [CrossRef] [PubMed]
12. McShane, R.; Arya, S.; Stewart, A.J.; Caie, P.D.; Bates, M. Prognostic features of the tumour microenvironment in oesophageal adenocarcinoma. *Biochim. Et Biophys. Acta (BBA)-Rev. Cancer* **2021**, *1876*, 188598. [CrossRef]
13. Doll, K.M.; Rademaker, A.; Sosa, J. Practical Guide to Surgical Data Sets: Surveillance, Epidemiology, and End Results (SEER) Database. *JAMA Surg.* **2018**, *153*, 588–589. [CrossRef]
14. Alsop, B.R.; Sharma, P. Esophageal Cancer. *Gastroenterol. Clin. North Am.* **2016**, *45*, 399–412. [CrossRef] [PubMed]
15. Popescu, B.; Popescu, C.R.; Grigore, R.; Mogoantă, C.A.; Ioniță, E.; Moculescu, C.; Berteşteanu, V.G. Morphology and morphopathology of hypopharyngo-esophageal cancer. *Romanian J. Morphol. Embryol.* **2012**, *53*, 243–248.
16. Mathieu, L.N.; Kanarek, N.F.; Tsai, H.-L.; Rudin, C.M.; Brock, M.V. Age and sex differences in the incidence of esophageal adenocarcinoma: Results from the Surveillance, Epidemiology, and End Results (SEER) Registry (1973–2008). *Dis. Esophagus* **2013**, *27*, 757–763. [CrossRef] [PubMed]
17. Greaves, M.; Maley, C. Clonal evolution in cancer. *Nature* **2012**, *481*, 306–313. [CrossRef]
18. Umar, S.B.; Fleischer, D.E. Esophageal cancer: Epidemiology, pathogenesis and prevention. *Nat. Clin. Pract. Gastroenterol. Hepatol.* **2008**, *5*, 517–526. [CrossRef]
19. Chen, S.B. Primary adenosquamous carcinoma of the esophagus. *World J. Gastroenterol.* **2013**, *19*, 8382–8390. [CrossRef]
20. Sasaki, Y.; Harada, M.; Kurosaki, S.; Shimada, Y.; Hayashi, M.; Kamiichi, H.; Kawamura, N.; Kajiyama, Y.; Yao, T. A case of adenosquamous carcinoma at the esophagogastric junction, initially diagnosed as collision carcinoma. *Nihon Shokakibyo Gakkai Zasshi* **2015**, *112*, 848–855.
21. Bombí, J.; Riverola, A.; Bordas, J.; Cardesa, A. Adenosquamous carcinoma of the esophagus. A case report. *Pathol. Res. Pract.* **1991**, *187*, 514–519; discussion 519–521. [CrossRef] [PubMed]
22. Orsatti, G.; Corvalan, A.; Sakurai, H.; Choi, H.S. Polypoid adenosquamous carcinoma of the esophagus with prominent spindle cells. Report of a case with immunohistochemical and ultrastructural studies. *Arch. Pathol. Lab. Med.* **1993**, *117*, 544–547. [PubMed]
23. Schizas, D.; Kapsampelis, P.; Mylonas, K. Adenosquamous Carcinoma of the Esophagus: A Literature Review. *J. Transl. Int. Med.* **2018**, *6*, 70–73. [CrossRef] [PubMed]
24. Chen, R.; Liu, Y.; Song, G.; Li, B.; Zhao, D.; Hua, Z.; Wang, X.; Li, J.; Hao, C.; Zhang, L.; et al. Effectiveness of one-time endoscopic screening programme in prevention of upper gastrointestinal cancer in China: A multicentre population-based cohort study. *Gut* **2021**, *70*, 251–260. [CrossRef]
25. Codipilly, D.C.; Qin, Y.; Dawsey, S.M.; Kisiel, J.; Topazian, M.; Ahlquist, D.; Lyer, P.G. Screening for esophageal squamous cell carcinoma: Recent advances. *Gastrointest. Endosc.* **2018**, *88*, 413–426. [CrossRef]
26. Lao-Sirieix, P.; Fitzgerald, R. Screening for oesophageal cancer. *Nat. Rev. Clin. Oncol.* **2012**, *9*, 278–287. [CrossRef]
27. Chen, K.-B.; Xuan, Y.; Lin, A.-J.; Guo, S.-H. Esophageal cancer detection based on classification of gastrointestinal CT images using improved Faster RCNN. *Comput. Methods Programs Biomed.* **2021**, *207*, 106172. [CrossRef]
28. Sun, Y.-H.; Lin, S.-W.; Chen, C.-H.; Liang, W.-Y.; Hsieh, C.-C. Adenosquamous Carcinoma of the Esophagus and Esophagogastric Junction: Clinical Manifestations and Treatment Outcomes. *J. Gastrointest. Surg.* **2015**, *19*, 1216–1222. [CrossRef]
29. Zhang, H.D.; Chen, C.G.; Gao, Y.Y.; Ma, Z.; Tang, P.; Duan, X.F.; Ren, P.; Yue, J.; Yu, Z. Primary esophageal adenosquamous carcinoma: A retrospective analysis of 24 cases. *Dis. Esophagus* **2014**, *27*, 783–789. [CrossRef]
30. Endo, H.; Koike, T.; Hatta, W.; Asanuma, K.; Uno, K.; Asano, N.; Imatani, A.; Watanabe, M.; Kato, K.; Masamune, A. Endoscopic Findings of Esophageal Adenosquamous Carcinoma Diagnosed by Endoscopic Mucosal Resection. *Case Rep. Gastroenterol.* **2019** *13*, 144–152. [CrossRef]
31. Liu, G.-Y.; Zhang, J.-X.; Rong, L.; Nian, W.-D.; Nian, B.-X.; Tian, Y. Esophageal superficial adenosquamous carcinoma resected by endoscopic submucosal dissection: A rare case report. *World J. Clin. Cases* **2021**, *9*, 1336–1342. [CrossRef] [PubMed]
32. Huang, Q.; Shi, J.; Sun, Q.; Fan, X.; Feng, A.; Wu, H.; Zhou, Q.; Yu, C.; Mashimo, H.; Lauwers, G.Y. Distal esophageal carcinomas in Chinese patients vary widely in histopathology, but adenocarcinomas remain rare. *Hum. Pathol.* **2012**, *43*, 2138–2148. [CrossRef] [PubMed]
33. Qian, H.; Ji, X.; Liu, C.; Dang, Y.; Li, X.; Zhang, G. Clinical Characteristics, Prognosis, and Nomogram for Esophageal Cancer Based on Adenosquamous Carcinoma: A SEER Database Analysis. *Front. Oncol.* **2021**, *11*, 603349. [CrossRef] [PubMed]
34. Yendamuri, S.; Malhotra, U.; Hennon, M.; Miller, A.; Groman, A.; Halloon, A.; Reid, M.E. Clinical characteristics of adenosquamous esophageal carcinoma. *J. Gastrointest. Oncol.* **2017**, *8*, 89–95. [CrossRef]
35. Chen, S.B.; Liu, D.; Chen, Y. Surgical resection for esophageal adenosquamous carcinoma: An analysis of 56 cases. *World J. Surg. Oncol.* **2022**, *20*, 143. [CrossRef]
36. Yachida, S.; Nakanishi, Y.; Shimoda, T.; Nimura, S.; Igaki, H.; Tachimori, Y.; Kato, H. Adenosquamous carcinoma of the esophagus. Clinicopathologic study of 18 cases. *Oncology* **2004**, *66*, 218–225. [CrossRef]

37. Mariette, C.; Piessen, G.; Triboulet, J. Therapeutic strategies in oesophageal carcinoma: Role of surgery and other modalities. *Lancet Oncol.* **2007**, *8*, 545–553. [CrossRef]
38. Smyth, E.C.; Lagergren, J.; Fitzgerald, R.C.; Lordick, F.; Shah, M.A.; Lagergren, P.; Cunningham, D. Oesophageal cancer. *Nat. Rev. Dis. Primers* **2017**, *3*, 17048. [CrossRef]
39. Demarest, C.T.; Chang, A. The Landmark Series: Multimodal Therapy for Esophageal Cancer. *Ann. Surg. Oncol.* **2021**, *28*, 3375–3382. [CrossRef]
40. Ohashi, S.; Miyamoto, S.; Kikuchi, O.; Goto, T.; Amanuma, Y.; Muto, M. Recent Advances From Basic and Clinical Studies of Esophageal Squamous Cell Carcinoma. *Gastroenterology* **2015**, *149*, 1700–1715. [CrossRef]
41. Ajani, J.A.; D'Amico, T.A.; Bentrem, D.J.; Chao, J.; Corvera, C.; Das, P.; Denlinger, C.S.; Enzinger, P.C.; Fanta, P.; Farjah, F.; et al. Esophageal and Esophagogastric Junction Cancers, Version 2.2019, NCCN Clinical Practice Guidelines in Oncology. *J. Natl. Compr. Canc. Netw.* **2019**, *17*, 855–883. [CrossRef] [PubMed]
42. Lu, Z.; Wang, J.; Shu, Y.; Liu, L.; Kong, L.; Yang, L.; Wang, B.; Sun, G.; Ji, Y.; Cao, G.; et al. Sintilimab versus placebo in combination with chemotherapy as first line treatment for locally advanced or metastatic oesophageal squamous cell carcinoma (ORIENT-15): Multicentre, randomised, double blind, phase 3 trial. *BMJ* **2022**, *377*, e068714. [CrossRef] [PubMed]
43. Sun, J.M.; Shen, L.; Shah, M.A.; Enzinger, P.; Adenis, A.; Doi, T.; Kojima, T.; Metges, J.P.; Li, Z.; Kim, S.B.; et al. Pembrolizumab plus chemotherapy versus chemotherapy alone for first-line treatment of advanced oesophageal cancer (KEYNOTE-590): A randomised, placebo-controlled, phase 3 study. *Lancet* **2021**, *398*, 759–771. [CrossRef] [PubMed]
44. Ni, P.-Z.; Yang, Y.-S.; Hu, W.-P.; Wang, W.-P.; Yuan, Y.; Chen, L.-Q. Primary adenosquamous carcinoma of the esophagus: An analysis of 39 cases. *J. Thorac. Dis.* **2016**, *8*, 2689–2696. [CrossRef] [PubMed]

Journal of Personalized Medicine

Review

Perineal Rectosigmoidectomy (Altemeier's Procedure) in the Treatment of Strangulated Rectal Prolapse: A Case Series and Literature Review

Ioannis Mantzoros [1,†], Aliki Brenta [1,*,†], Aikaterini-Antonia Bourtzinakou [1], Ourania Kontaxi [1], Georgios Gemousakakis [1], Nikolaos Antoniou [2], Stefanos Bitsianis [1], Efstathios Kotidis [1], Dimitrios Kyziridis [1], Orestis Ioannidis [1], Ourania Kerasidou [1], Anna Gkiouliava [3], Manousos Pramateftakis [1] and Stamatios Aggelopoulos [1]

1 4th Department of Surgery, General Hospital of Thessaloniki "G. Papanikolaou", School of Medicine, Faculty of Health Science, Aristotle University of Thessaloniki, 541 24 Thessaloniki, Greece; imantzoros@auth.gr (I.M.); katerbourtzi@gmail.com (A.-A.B.); ourania.kontaxi@nhs.net (O.K.); ggemous@auth.gr (G.G.); sbits@auth.gr (S.B.); skotidis@auth.gr (E.K.); dkyzir@auth.gr (D.K.); iorestis@auth.gr (O.I.); koura@auth.gr (O.K.); mpramate@auth.gr (M.P.); saggelopoulos@auth.gr (S.A.)
2 2nd Department of Surgery, General Hospital of Thessaloniki "G. Gennimatas", School of Medicine, Faculty of Health Science, Aristotle University of Thessaloniki, 541 24 Thessaloniki, Greece; nantoniou@auth.gr
3 Department of Anesthesiology and Intensive Care, School of Medicine, Faculty of Health Science, Aristotle University of Thessaloniki, 541 24 Thessaloniki, Greece; annagkio@gmail.com
* Correspondence: alikibrenta@gmail.com; Tel.: +30-694-577-9808
† These authors contributed equally to this work.

Abstract: Background: Rectal prolapse (RP) predominantly affects women over the age of 50 and presents as mucosal, internal, or full thickness prolapse. Strangulated rectal prolapse requires immediate medical intervention, and surgical treatment options include both abdominal and perineal approaches. We aim to present a case series of perineal rectosigmoidectomy performed urgently due to strangulation and argue that Altemeier's procedure is the preferred method for treating strangulated rectal prolapse. Methods: Perineal rectosigmoidectomy, particularly Altemeier's procedure, is effective for incarcerated cases. Altemeier's procedure with diverting ileostomy was used in all three patients. Results: All patients were successfully treated, with no recurrence of prolapse and stool incontinence. Conclusions: Altemeier's procedure is ideal for the treatment of strangulated rectal prolapse.

Keywords: rectal prolapse; incarcerated; perineal rectosigmoidectomy; Altemeier's procedure

1. Introduction

Rectal prolapse is an uncommon condition that occurs more frequently in women after the fifth decade. A strangulated (or incarcerated) rectal prolapse refers to a condition in which the full thickness prolapsing rectum cannot be manually repositioned. Unlike reducible prolapse, which can be pushed back into place, a strangulated prolapse remains extended, leading to mucosal or full thickness ischemia and resulting in septic complications. This condition requires immediate surgical intervention [1,2]. Surgical treatment options include both abdominal and perineal approaches [3]. Altemeier's procedure is considered the preferred technique for treating strangulated rectal prolapse [1–3]. Here, we aim to present three cases of strangulated rectal prolapse treated at our hospital with Altemeier's procedure, along with a literature review.

2. Description of Surgical Technique

Rectal prolapse can manifest clinically as mucosal prolapse (partial or pseudoprolapse), internal prolapse (rectal intussusception), or full thickness prolapse.

Various techniques have been proposed for the treatment of rectal prolapse, including abdominal approaches (Ripstein, Wells, and Orr-Loygue) and perineal procedures (Altemeier, Delorme, and Thiersch). Additionally, laparoscopic and open techniques have been developed, with or without the use of mesh. The choice of surgical method should be tailored to each patient's specific condition and the extent of rectal prolapse. Perineal procedures are often performed under regional anesthesia. They are associated with lower morbidity and mortality, although they may have higher recurrence rates. Altemeier's procedure typically involves perineal rectosigmoidectomy combined with anterior levatorplasty, which addresses the separation of the levator muscles seen in this condition, theoretically improving fecal continence [3–5]. Preoperatively, the large intestine is mechanically cleansed one day one day before surgery. The patient is positioned in the prone jackknife or Lloyd-Davies position, and a Foley catheter is inserted immediately after caudal anesthesia. Patients receive routine antibiotic prophylaxis.

During surgery, the prolapsed rectal mucosa is gradually grasped with Babcock or Allis clamps until the full-thickness prolapse is exposed, with eversion of the dental line. A circumferential incision is made 1.5 cm above the dentate line to achieve tissue dissection. The anterior peritoneal reflection is then incised to access the peritoneal cavity. The mesentery of the rectum and sigmoid colon is systematically clamped and ligated, and the mesenteric vessels are coagulated before removing the excess bowel. Optionally, the surgeon may perform anterior and posterior levatorplasty using separate 2-0 non-absorbable sutures to address the levator ani diastasis. The colon is then excised, and a coloanal anastomosis is created using interrupted sutures or staples. A protective ileostomy may also be performed, depending on the viability of the anastomosis.

3. Case Report

We present three cases of strangulated rectal prolapse using Altemeier's procedure in an emergency setting:

Case 1: A 62-year-old male, a long-distance swimmer, presented with severe pain and a full-thickness incarcerated prolapse, showing signs of ischemia (Figure 1). Symptoms had begun earlier that day. The patient had a history of three previous hemorrhoidectomies and a lateral internal sphincterotomy for an anal fissure. The prolapse occurred five hours prior during defecation. An Altemeier procedure with a prophylactic ileostomy was performed under epidural anesthesia. The postoperative course was uneventful (Clavien–Dindo Classification: Grade 0), and the patient was discharged five days later. Ileostomy reversal was performed six months later. No levatorplasty was performed.

Case 2: An 83-year-old female presented with a 20 cm full-thickness rectal prolapse, which she had been managing for the past five years. Initially, the prolapse was mechanically reducible, but over time, it progressively increased in length and became strangulated eight hours before admission (Figure 2). The patient had a history of three vaginal deliveries. Inflammatory markers were within normal range. Conservative treatments, including positioning the patient in the Trendelenburg position and applying granulated sugar topically, were attempted but unsuccessful. A rectosigmoidectomy was required, and an Altemeier procedure with a prophylactic ileostomy was performed. She was discharged seven days later with no postoperative complications (Clavien–Dindo Classification: Grade 0). No levatorplasty was performed.

Case 3: A 43-year-old female with a prolonged history of psychiatric institutionalization presented with pain and an incarcerated rectal prolapse that had worsened over the previous five days (Figure 3). The patient had a history of chronic constipation but no pregnancies. Altemeier's procedure with a prophylactic ileostomy was performed under epidural anesthesia. On the fourth postoperative day, the patient developed sepsis due to aspiration pneumonia, presenting with fever and abnormal auscultatory findings. She recovered with antibiotic treatment (Clavien–Dindo Classification: Grade II) and was discharged on the fifteenth postoperative day. No levatorplasty was performed.

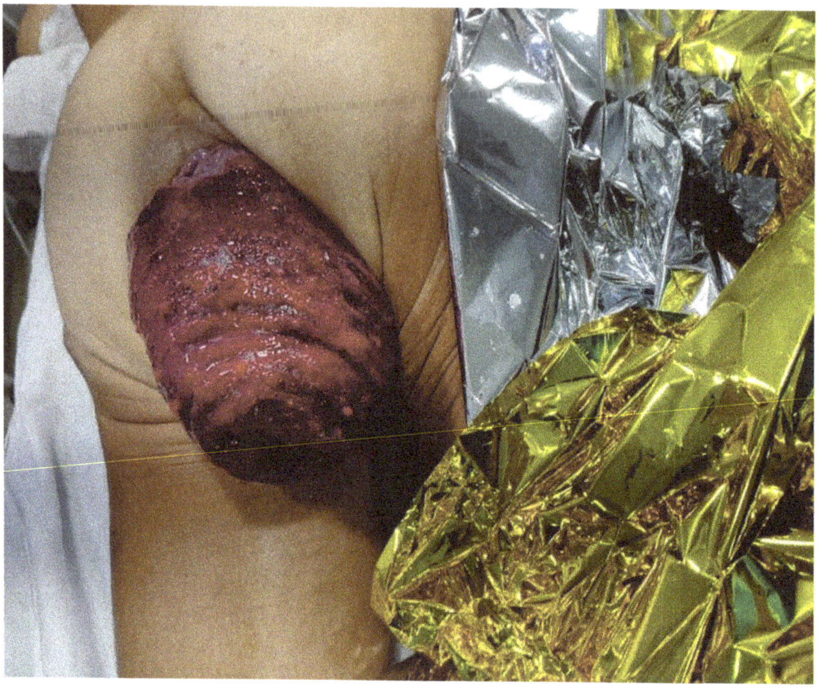

Figure 1. A 62-year-old male with incarcerated rectal prolapse with mucosal necrosis.

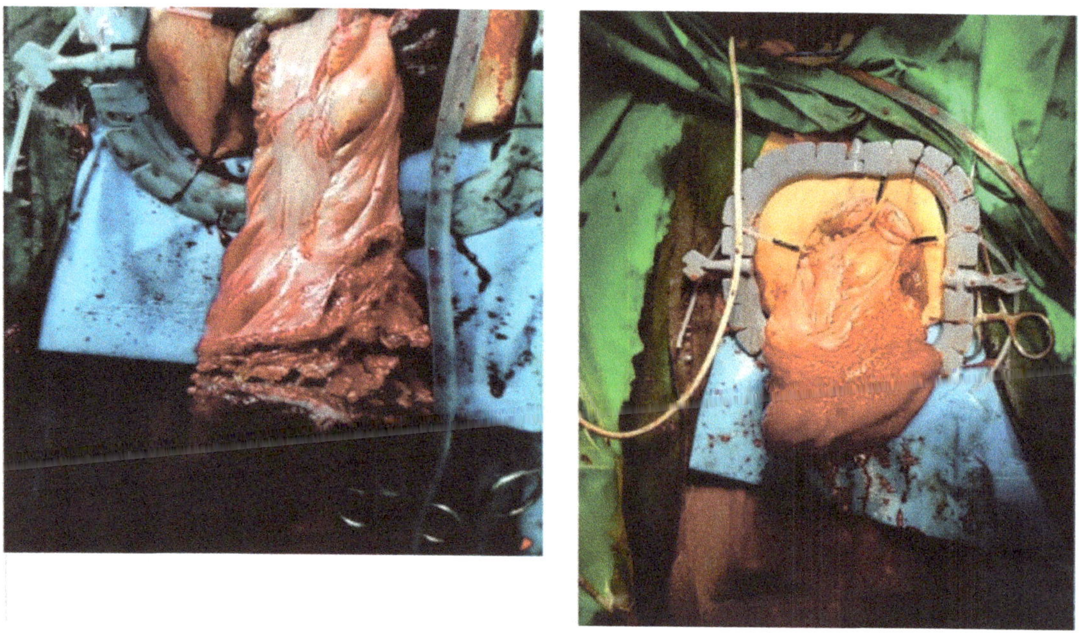

Figure 2. An 83-year-old female with large incarcerated prolapse.

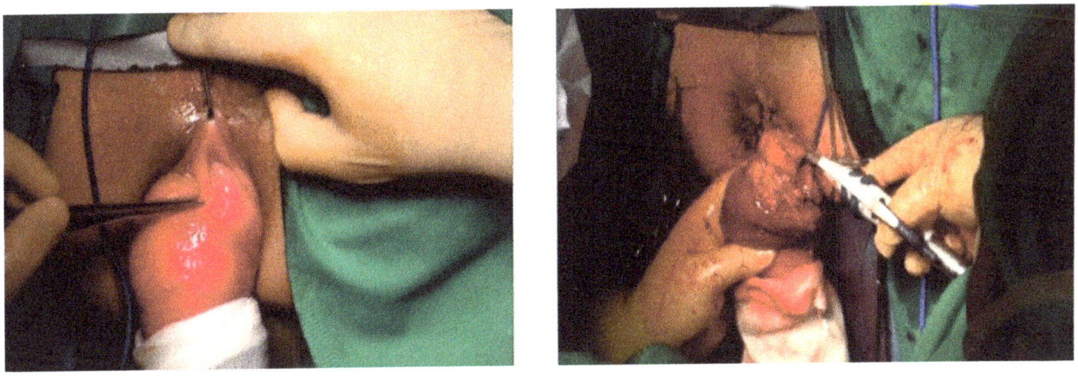

Figure 3. A 43-year-old female with a psychiatric background with pain and an incarcerated rectal prolapse.

4. Follow-Up

Patients were scheduled for follow-up visits at 2 weeks and 3, 6, and 12 months after ileostomy reversal to ensure proper monitoring. Additional follow-up visits were scheduled at 24 and 36 months. Prolapse recurrence was assessed clinically, and incontinence was measured using the Cleveland Clinic Incontinence Score after ileostomy reversal. All three patients reported complete continence within the first 6 months after surgery. None of the patients experienced a recurrence of prolapse or stool incontinence during the follow-up period. To prevent incontinence, we advised all patients to perform Kegel pelvic floor exercises three times daily after undergoing Altemeier's procedure.

5. Discussion

The prevalence of external rectal prolapse in the general population is less than 0.5%, with the majority of patients being women over the age of 50 [6]. Although the exact etiology of rectal prolapse is unknown, the most widely accepted theory, supported by defecography studies, is rectoanal intussusception [2]. Several factors appear to contribute, including multiple childbirths, the deterioration of the rectoanal inhibitory reflex, intermittent high-pressure rectal motor activity, anorectal sensory disorders, and pudendal neuropathy [1]. Rectal prolapse is more common among elderly patients, those with a history of vaginal births, chronic psychiatric disorders, and Ehlers–Danlos syndrome type 2. The literature associates rectal prolapse with age, multiparity, pelvic floor dysfunction, and perineal injury. Anatomical abnormalities, such as loose attachment of the rectum to the sacrum, lax lateral ligaments, a redundant sigmoid colon, a patulous anus, and diastasis of the levator ani muscles, are also linked to the development of rectal prolapse [3].

Initially, the prolapse may descend during defecation or straining but retract spontaneously afterward. Patients often report feeling a mass or lump that needs to be manually repositioned after bowel movements. Some may experience fecal incontinence caused by the prolapse or a persistent sensation of moisture and mucus discharge in the perineal area. A minor or spontaneously retractable prolapse can eventually progress to a chronically prolapsed rectum, requiring manual reduction. Over time, the rectal mucosa can become thickened or ulcerated, leading to significant bleeding. In rare cases, the prolapsed segment may become trapped below the anal sphincter, necessitating urgent surgical intervention.

According to the latest WSES-AAST (World Society of Emergency Medicine-American Association for the Surgery of Trauma) guidelines, the initial management of uncomplicated rectal prolapse involves non-operative methods, such as submucosal injection of epinephrine or hyaluronidase, rectal insertion of hypertonic dextrose- or mannitol-treated gauze, and elastic band wrapping, typically performed in a mildly sedated patient positioned in the Trendelenburg position. Strangulation of rectal prolapse is an uncommon complication, occurring in 2–4% of cases. In such instances, or when complications like hemodynamic instability, peritonitis, gangrene, or perforation arise, prompt surgical intervention through either perineal or abdominal approaches is recommended [4].

Various techniques exist for rectal prolapse repair, including abdominal and perineal approaches. Perineal surgery is associated with a higher recurrence rate, while abdominal surgery has a lower recurrence rate but a higher mortality risk and may be associated with complications such as impotence and infertility [5]. Abdominal approaches include suture rectopexy with or without resection, posterior mesh rectopexy, anterior sling (Ripstein procedure) rectopexy, and laparoscopic rectopexy [2]. Surgical options are more challenging in cases of incarceration due to the increased risk of anastomotic complications from bowel edema [6]. In cases where the bowel is irreducible and ischemic, excision may be required, which is typically achieved through a perineal approach [7]. The goal of surgery is to excise the affected bowel and any redundant tissue to prevent recurrence, although this can be difficult to assess, particularly when dealing with thickened, edematous tissues in strangulated cases.

The two preferred techniques for managing strangulated prolapse are mucosal resection with muscular plication (Delorme) and perineal rectosigmoidectomy (Altemeier), with younger, healthier individuals potentially benefiting from a transabdominal approach. Delorme's procedure is suitable when ischemia is confined to the mucosa. In our series, all the patients presented with strangulated full-thickness rectal prolapse. In these cases, Delorme's procedure, although less risky in older adult patients, is not problem-solving. For rectal prolapse repair, a perineal approach is generally favored over abdominal surgery, particularly for older or medically complex patients, as it results in fewer postoperative complications. One key advantage of this method is that it can be performed under epidural anesthesia, making Altemeier's procedure especially appropriate for older patients with significant comorbidities. Ramanujan and Venkatesh underscored the effectiveness of perineal rectosigmoidectomy by successfully treating 8 older adult women among 70 cases over an 8-year period [8,9]. Despite its higher recurrence rate, the perineal approach is often preferred in older patients with comorbidities due to its lower complication rates and better patient tolerance. It is also a viable option in irreducible cases requiring emergency surgery.

Postoperative morbidity following perineal rectosigmoidectomy has been reported to be low, with complications occurring in only 10–12% of cases. The most serious complication, anastomotic leak, is more common in cases of incarcerated prolapse due to the presence of edema, which complicates anastomosis and increases the risk of breakdown. The risk of anastomotic leak in elective rectosigmoidectomy is 2–6%, but this rises to 25% in cases of incarceration [2]. Factors such as inadequate perfusion, edema, tension, and elevated intraluminal pressure contribute to the risk of anastomotic leaks, with an incidence of 10–15% in high-risk areas like the rectum and 5–10% elsewhere [10,11]. While fecal diversion can reduce the risk of leak, it does not eliminate it entirely.

Two recent studies found partial anastomotic dehiscence and leaks in a small number of patients undergoing perineal rectosigmoidectomy with or without diversion [12,13]. A case series reported two patients with incarcerated prolapse, with one requiring diversion due to concerns about mucosal necrosis; both had uneventful post-operative courses [6]. This suggests that anastomotic leaks are multifactorial and may still occur despite diversion [14–16], Thus, the decision to use adjunctive ileostomy should be customized according to the patient's individual condition, overall health, and the specific circumstances of the prolapse. In our case series, a diverting loop ileostomy was performed in all three cases, and none of the patients experienced dehiscence. We used a trephine loop ileostomy technique, accessing the abdominal cavity through a small incision, which avoided the need for a full laparotomy. This approach is minimally invasive, and spinal anesthesia was sufficient. Spinal anesthesia was preferred, as it avoids further strain on already compromised patients, especially given the presence of bowel strangulation and serious comorbidities. Even when ileostomies are performed under general anesthesia, spinal anesthesia helps with postoperative pain management. Thus, the ability to perform this perineal technique under spinal anesthesia remains advantageous. The decision for stool diversion was particularly important considering the patients' poor nutritional status, as the procedure was performed on an emergency basis in older adult patients with nutritional and psychiatric challenges. Moreover, this method facilitates the subsequent reversal of the ileostomy and the creation of an ileo-colonic anastomosis at a later stage.

Stool continence is another critical factor. Our patients reported intermittent incontinence due to constant bowel irritation before surgery. Stool incontinence in rectal prolapse results from the disruption and weakening of the anal sphincters and pelvic floor muscles, as well as nerve damage and irritation from chronic prolapse. These factors impair the ability to control stool passage and maintain continence. In all cases, continence was restored within 3 to 6 months after the procedure.

Many studies have evaluated continence following elective Altemeier's procedure. The results of these studies are presented in Table 1. For this reason, perineal rectosigmoidectomy has been modified with the addition of levatorplasty. The main reasons for adding levatorplasty are to address the high preoperative rate of fecal incontinence and to prevent recurrent prolapse. Chun et al. reported recurrence rates of 7.7% with levatorplasty compared with 20.6% without it [17]. This procedure improves anal continence by restoring the anorectal angle and offers additional benefits, such as lower short-term recurrence rates and a longer recurrence-free interval. However, other studies suggest that levatorplasty may not add significant value when combined with Altemeier's procedure [18–21]. As a team, we opted not to perform levatorplasty in some cases because the levator ani muscle is often already weakened, and attempts to restore it might further compromise its integrity, potentially worsening incontinence. Bananzadeh et al. compared the outcomes of Altemeier's procedure performed with and without posterior levatorplasty [22]. In their retrospective study, they found no significant reduction in fecal incontinence with posterior levatorplasty. The pathophysiology of incontinence related to rectal prolapse involves pelvic muscle relaxation, pudendal nerve paralysis, and sphincter relaxation. Therefore, we believe that postoperative muscle training, biofeedback, and nerve stimulation may be more beneficial than levatorplasty in improving patient outcomes. These treatments have been used successfully for incontinence improvement in the past [23–25].

The relationship between sphincterotomy in one of our patients and rectal prolapse is not definitively proven. The internal sphincter contributes approximately 25–30% to the continence mechanism [19,20]. In the first case, in which the patient had previously undergone internal sphincterotomy, attempting to surgically restore the internal sphincter's anatomy would likely not have significantly affected the patient's continence. Our approach is to follow up postoperatively and, in cases of severe incontinence, assess the sphincter mechanism using manometry, endoscopic ultrasound, and MRI, and then decide whether anatomical restoration is warranted. The authors suggest that internal sphincter restoration would not benefit neither the continence nor the recurrence rates.

Recurrence rates are generally higher with the perineal approach (up to 20% after Altemeier's procedure and up to 30% after Delorme's) than with the abdominal approach [16]. According to the literature [7], several technical factors play a significant role. Kim et al. found that patients who underwent stapled anastomosis had a significantly higher recurrence rate than those with hand-sewn anastomosis [26]. Additionally, patients with a shorter length of resected tissue were at greater risk of relapse than those with longer resections. Furthermore, having a prolapse for more than six months prior to surgery was associated with a higher risk of recurrence, although this increase was not statistically significant [26]. Several studies indicate that recurrence is linked to factors such as the length of bowel resected, the surgeon's level of experience, and the type of anastomosis performed [19,27,28]. In our opinion, attempting to repair the internal sphincter may compromise the sphincter mechanism more than it would benefit continence or reduce recurrence. While the literature identifies various factors contributing to recurrence, many of these are unrelated to the sphincter mechanism. Thus, we believe that repairing the internal sphincter would not significantly reduce the risk of recurrence. Recurrence following

Altemeier's procedure typically depends on technical fouls, and the majority of recurrences present in the first year following the operation. The most common cause of recurrence is excision of inadequate sigmoid resection. In these cases, the spare mobile sigmoid colon prolapses again and results in early recurrence. In our series, the follow up was 36 months, which is considered a sufficiently safe time frame to make conclusions about recurrences related or unrelated to technical errors.

All techniques for the restoration of rectal prolapse, whether perineal or abdominal, carry recurrence rates ranging between 0–30% [16,29,30]. Altemeier's procedure does not directly affect the internal sphincter or pelvic floor muscles, but it can alleviate constipation by removing the redundant sigmoid colon. However, the underlying causes of prolapse often remain, and perineal techniques are generally associated with higher—though acceptable—recurrence rates. The literature links recurrence more to technical factors than physiological ones [19,27,28]. It is important to note that our case series involves strangulated rectal prolapse with ischemic bowel, which made the abdominal approach unsuitable. Our primary goal was to salvage the remaining colon, as Altemeier's procedure was performed as an emergency. In this context, recurrence was a secondary concern.

Incorporating laparoscopy into the perineal approach for rectal prolapse is an innovative technique. It aids in evaluating the length of the sigmoid, facilitates colonic mobilization, and ensures thorough excision of redundant bowel. By directly assessing bowel length and redundancy, laparoscopy helps the surgeon determine the necessary extent of resection [15]. However, laparoscopy is contraindicated in cases of strangulation, as attempting to reduce ischemic or necrotic bowel back into the abdominal cavity can lead to infection spread and sepsis due to compromised tissue.

Most of the articles published regarding Altemeier's procedure, as shown in Table 1, either do not specify the type of prolapse (whether chronic or acutely complicated by incarceration and strangulation) or refer to elective surgeries. In the context of incarcerated prolapse, surgical treatment options are extremely limited, and the literature suggests that the ideal approach is Altemeier's procedure [8,31]. Altemeier's procedure is typically preferred for patients with comorbidities because it can be performed under spinal or regional anesthesia, avoiding the need for laparotomy and allowing for quicker recovery and earlier mobilization [21]. Altemeier's procedure is typically preferred for patients with comorbidities because it can be performed under spinal or regional anesthesia, avoiding the need for laparotomy and allowing for quicker recovery and earlier mobilization [18,21,27,32,33]. By contrast, abdominal repair requires general anesthesia and poses the risk of pelvic adhesions, which may compromise fertility in young women and cause impotence in men. There is also the risk of anastomotic leakage if a resection rectopexy is performed, though resections are now rarely performed [34]. The minimally invasive nature of Altemeier's procedure and its ability to be repeated without significantly increasing the risk of complications make it an ideal choice for patients with strangulated prolapse and those with comorbidities [21].

Most studies focus on patients undergoing rectosigmoidectomy in an elective setting, as strangulation is a rare complication. When the prolapsed bowel becomes incarcerated or gangrenous and cannot be repositioned using standard methods, surgical intervention becomes an emergency, as was the case for our patients. Immediate surgery is crucial to prevent compromising bowel viability, as gangrene significantly increases the risk of complications and mortality [5]. Altemeier's procedure remains the gold standard for treating incarcerated prolapse, surpassing abdominal approaches since necrotic bowel cannot be returned to the abdominal cavity and requires full-thickness resection. Additionally, the perineal approach avoids the use of mesh, reducing the risk of infection at a new site. As noted earlier, perineal procedures are particularly suitable for high-risk patients. An abdominal surgery to remove the affected segment would likely require a colostomy and would carry higher risks for these already compromised patients.

Apart from those presented in Table 1, there are several case reports in the literature regarding the treatment of strangulated prolapse using Altemeier's technique. Voulimeneas et al. reported a complicated case of gangrenous rectal prolapse treated with Altemeier's procedure and prophylactic ileostomy [5], while Nguyen et al. successfully treated two cases of irreducible incarcerated prolapse with perineal rectosigmoidectomy, one of which required fecal diversion [35]. Cernuda et al. found no recurrence of prolapse six months after performing Altemeier's procedure with loop ileostomy [9]. Recent case reports also demonstrate positive outcomes in treating strangulated rectal prolapse using Altemeier's technique, further underscoring its effectiveness [36–38].

Our study, while limited by its retrospective design and small sample size, addresses the rare emergency of rectal prolapse complicated by strangulation. The design of an RCT or a meta-analysis is difficult, considering the rarity of strangulated cases. The available literature on this condition is sparse, and most studies in our literature review focus on elective Altemeier's procedures. For this reason, our sample is very specific, and to our knowledge, there are no systematic reviews or larger studies regarding the management of strangulated rectal prolapse specifically. Furthermore, since our cases involved strangulated prolapse, abdominal procedures were not a viable option, precluding a comparison of approaches. When strangulation and ischemic bowel are present, there is an indication for Altemeier's technique [1,2,5–9,31]. The goal of this study was to present the outcomes of our case series involving three patients who underwent urgent Altemeier's procedures due to strangulation. There is limited evidence regarding outcomes with other techniques in cases of strangulation, but individual case reports support our view that Altemeier's technique is the ideal treatment for this rare emergency.

Table 1. Literature review of results after Altemeier's Procedure.

Authors	N	Study	Levatorplasty	Incarcerated # (%)	Mortality # (%)	Continence %	Constipation %	Recurrence # (%)	Follow-Up, Months
Johansen et al., 1993 [39]	20	Not stated	No	No	1 (5)	21	Not stated	0	26
Ramanujam et al., 1994 [40]	72	Not stated	No	9 (13)	0	67	Not stated	4 (6)	120
Deen et al., 1994 [41]	10	Prospective	No	No	0	80	Not stated	1 (10)	18
Agachan et al., 1997 [29]	32	Retrospective	No	No	0	+	Not stated	4 (13)	30
Takesue et al., 1999 [31]	10	Not stated	Yes (7)	Not stated	0	+	Not stated	0	42
Kim et al. 1999 [28]	183	Retrospective	No	Not stated	Not stated	53	61 (+)	29 (16)	47
Kimmins et al. 2001 [21]	63	Retrospective	Yes (29)	4 (6)	0	87	31.7	4 (6.3)	21
Zbar et al., 2002 [42]	80	Retrospective	Yes	Not stated	0	100	Not stated	3 (3.8)	22
Chun et al., 2004 [17]	109	Retrospective	Yes	Not stated	0	100	Not stated	18 (16.5)	29
Habr gama et al., 2006 [43]	44	Retrospective	Yes	Not stated	0	85	Not stated	3 (7.1)	49
Boccasanta et al., 2006 [44]	40	RTC	Yes	Not stated	Not stated	100	Not stated	5 (12.5)	28
Altomare et al., 2009 [16]	93	Retrospective	No	Not stated	0	47	+	5 (25)	41
Cirocco WC 2010 [27]	103	Not stated	Yes	Not stated	0	83	94 (+)	0	43
Ris et al., 2011 [18]	60	Not stated	Yes	Not stated	1.6	62	Not stated	(14)	48
Senapati et al., 2013 [33]	102	RTC	Not stated	Not stated	(2)	(+)	Not stated	24 (24)	60
Kim et al., 2014 [26]	63	Retrospective	Yes (33)	Not stated	(1.6)	Not stated	Not stated	8 (12.7)	33
Trompeto et al., 2019 [45]	43	Retrospective	Yes (21)	Not stated	0	No change	(+)	(40)	49
Boccasanta et al., 2021 [30]	130	Retrospective	Yes	Not stated	4 (3.1)	(+)	(+)	27 (20.8)	82

#: absolute number; (+): favorable results but no specified percentage.

6. Conclusions

In conclusion, perineal rectosigmoidectomy stands as a viable treatment option for incarcerated and strangulated rectal prolapse, offering low mortality and acceptable recurrence rates. The literature, as well as our experience, emphasizes the importance of early surgical intervention, particularly in cases of strangulated rectal prolapse complicated by necrosis. This underscores the value of perineal proctosigmoidectomy in addressing this rare surgical emergency. Overall, Altemeier's procedure is ideal for the treatment of strangulated rectal prolapse.

Author Contributions: Conceptualization, I.M.; methodology, A.B.; validation, E.K., O.I., M.P. and S.A.; formal analysis, D.K.; investigation, A.B., A.-A.B., O.K. (Ourania Kontaxi), N.A.; resources, I.M. and N.A.; data curation, I.M., G.G. and D.K.; writing—original draft preparation, A.B., O.K. (Ourania Kontaxi), G.G., N.A., O.K. (Ourania Kerasidou) and A.G.; writing—review and editing, I.M., S.B., E.K., O.I. and M.P.; visualization, A.B., A.-A.B. and G.G.; supervision, I.M. and S.A.; project administration, S.B., A.G. and S.A. All authors have read and agreed to the published version of the manuscript.

Funding: This research received no external funding.

Institutional Review Board Statement: The study was conducted in accordance with the Declaration of Helsinki, and approved by the the Institutional Review Board of G. Papanikolaou General Hospital(protocol code 911 and date of approval is 30 July 2024), extraordinary meeting of commission (protocol code 10,subject 26, and date of approval is 29 July 2024).

Informed Consent Statement: Informed consent was obtained from all participants involved in the study and all participants agreed to publish.

Data Availability Statement: No new data were created or analyzed in this study. Data sharing is not applicable to this article.

Conflicts of Interest: The authors declare no conflicts of interest.

References

1. Ben Ameur, H.; Rejab, H.; Beyrouti, M.I. Altemeier operation for recurred and strangulated rectal prolapse. *Indian J. Surg.* **2013**, *75* (Suppl. S1), 224–226. [CrossRef] [PubMed]
2. Sipahi, M.; Arslan, E.; Börekçi, H.; Aytekin, F.Ö.; Külah, B.; Banlı, O. Perineal rectosigmoidectomy for incarcerated rectal prolapse (Altemeier's procedure). *Ulus. Cerrahi Derg.* **2015**, *32*, 217–220. [CrossRef]
3. Goldstein, S.D.; Maxwell, P.J., 4th. Rectal prolapse. *Clin. Colon. Rectal Surg.* **2011**, *24*, 39–45. [CrossRef]
4. Ahmadinejad, M.; Farsi, Y.; Bahr, M.H.; Bozorgmehr, R.; Soltanian, A.; Zebarjadi Bagherpour, J. A case report of largest rectal prolapse in the literature successfully treated with Altemeier's procedure. *Ann. Med. Surg.* **2022**, *80*, 104231. [CrossRef] [PubMed]
5. Voulimeneas, I.; Antonopoulos, C.; Alifierakis, E.; Ioannides, P. Perineal rectosigmoidectomy for gangrenous rectal prolapse. *Word J. Gastroenterol.* **2010**, *16*, 2689–2691. [CrossRef] [PubMed]
6. Chaouch, M.A.; Sallem, R.; Jabra, S.B.; Chedly, E.; Gafsi, B.; Noomen, F. Altemeier procedure for strangulated rectal prolapse: A case report. *Int. J. Surg. Case Rep.* **2024**, *114*, 109216. [CrossRef]
7. Kraiem, I.; Kellil, T.; Chaouch, M.A.; Korbi, I.; Zouari, K. Strangled rectal prolapse in young adults: A case report. *Ann. Med. Surg.* **2022**, *55*, 33–35. [CrossRef] [PubMed]
8. Ramanujam, P.S.; Venkatesh, K.S. Management of acute incarcerated rectal prolapse. *Dis. Colon. Rectum.* **1992**, *35*, 1154–1156. [CrossRef] [PubMed]
9. Cernuda, R.B.; Ángel, J.P.; Fernández, N.T.; Sánchez-Farpón, J.H.; Pérez, J.A. Perineal Rectosigmoidectomy (Altemeier Procedure) as Treatment of Strangulated Rectal Prolapse. *J. Gastrointest. Surg.* **2016**, *20*, 2102–2103. [CrossRef] [PubMed]
10. Yamamoto, T.; Hyakudomi, R.; Takai, K.; Taniura, T.; Uchida, Y.; Ishitobi, K.; Hirahara, N.; Tajima, Y. Altemeier perineal rectosigmoidectomy with indocyanine green fluorescence imaging for a female adolescent with complete rectal prolapse: A case report. *World J. Clin. Cases.* **2021**, *9*, 847–853. [CrossRef]
11. Guyton, K.L.; Hyman, N.H.; Alverdy, J.C. Prevention of Perioperative Anastomotic Healing Complications: Anastomotic Stricture and Anastomotic Leak. *Adv. Surg.* **2016**, *50*, 129–141. [CrossRef]
12. Abdelhamid, A.F.; Elsheikh, M.; Hablus, M.A.; Barakat, H.; Youssef, T. Perineal proctosigmoidectomy with covering ileostomy is an acceptable and safe procedure for irreducible rectal prolapse. *Austin J. Surg.* **2019**, *6*, 1188.
13. Alwahid, M.; Knight, S.R.; Wadhawan, H.; Campbell, K.L.; Ziyaie, D.; Koch, S.M.P. Perineal rectosigmoidectomy for rectal prolapse-the preferred procedure for the unfit elderly patient? 10 years experience from a UK tertiary centre. *Tech. Coloproctol.* **2019**, *23*, 1065–1072. [CrossRef] [PubMed]
14. Biegel, C.; Brock, S.; Porter, J.; Kim, D. A modified perineal approach for the management of strangulated rectal prolapse: A case report. *Int. J. Surg. Case Rep.* **2023**, *109*, 108504. [CrossRef] [PubMed]
15. Al-Ameen, W.M.; Privitera, A.; Al-Ayed, A.; Sabr, K. Laparoscopic-Assisted Altemeier's Procedure for Recurrent Strangulated Rectal Prolapse: A Case Report. *Am. J. Case Rep.* **2016**, *17*, 827–829. [CrossRef] [PubMed]
16. Altomare, D.F.; Binda, G.; Ganio, E.; De Nardi, P.; Giamundo, P.; Pescatori, M.; Rectal Prolapse Study Group. Long-term outcome of Altemeier's procedure for rectal prolapse. *Dis. Colon. Rectum.* **2009**, *52*, 698–703. [CrossRef] [PubMed]
17. Chun, S.W.; Pikarsky, A.J.; You, S.Y.; Gervaz, P.; Efron, J.; Weiss, E.; Nogueras, J.J.; Wexner, S.D. Perineal rectosigmoidectomy for rectal prolapse: Role of levatorplasty. *Tech. Coloproctol.* **2004**, *8*, 3–8; discussion 8–9. [CrossRef] [PubMed]

18. Ris, F.; Colin, J.F.; Chilcott, M.; Remue, C.; Jamart, J.; Kartheuser, A. Altemeier's procedure for rectal prolapse: Analysis of long-term outcome in 60 patients. *Color. Dis.* **2012**, *14*, 1106–1111. [CrossRef] [PubMed]
19. Glasgow, S.C.; Birnbaum, E.H.; Kodner, I.J.; Fleshman, J.W., Jr.; Dietz, D.W. Recurrence and quality of life following perineal proctectomy for rectal prolapse. *J. Gastrointest. Surg.* **2008**, *12*, 1446–1451. [CrossRef]
20. Ding, J.H.; Canedo, J.; Lee, S.H.; Kalaskar, S.N.; Rosen, L.; Wexner, S.D. Perineal rectosigmoidectomy for primary and recurrent rectal prolapse: Are the results comparable the second time? *Dis. Colon. Rectum.* **2012**, *55*, 666–670. [CrossRef]
21. Kimmins, M.H.; Evetts, B.K.; Isler, J.; Billingham, R. The Altemeier repair: Outpatient treatment of rectal prolapse. *Dis. Colon. Rectum.* **2001**, *44*, 565–570. [CrossRef] [PubMed]
22. Bananzadeh, A.; Shariat-Razavi, H.; Khodaei, S. Outcome of Fecal Incontinence in Patients with Rectal Prolapse Undergoing the Altemeier Procedure with or without Posterior Levatorplasty. *J. Coloproctol.* **2021**, *41*, 52–57. [CrossRef]
23. Norton, C.; Whitehead, W.E.; Bliss, D.Z.; Harari, D.; Lang, J.; Conservative Management of Fecal Incontinence in Adults Committee of the International Consultation on Incontinence. Management of fecal incontinence in adults. *Neurourol. Urodyn.* **2010**, *29*, 199–206. [CrossRef] [PubMed]
24. Norton, C.; Cody, J.D.; Hosker, G. Biofeedback and/or sphincter exercises for the treatment of faecal incontinence in adults. *Cochrane Database Syst. Rev.* **2012**, *2012*, CD002111. [CrossRef] [PubMed] [PubMed Central]
25. Vonthein, R.; Heimerl, T.; Schwandner, T. Electrical stimulation and biofeedback for the treatment of fecal incontinence: A systematic review. *Int. J. Color. Dis.* **2013**, *28*, 1567–1577. [CrossRef] [PubMed]
26. Kim, M.; Reibetanz, J.; Schlegel, N.; Krajinovic, K.; Köstler, H.; Germer, C.T.; Isbert, C. Recurrence after perineal rectosigmoidectomy: When and why? *Color. Dis.* **2014**, *16*, 920–924. [CrossRef]
27. Cirocco, W.C. The Altemeier procedure for rectal prolapse: An operation for all ages. *Dis. Colon. Rectum.* **2010**, *53*, 1618–1623. [CrossRef] [PubMed]
28. Kim, D.S.; Tsang, C.B.; Wong, W.D.; Lowry, A.C.; Goldberg, S.M.; Madoff, R.D. Complete rectal prolapse: Evolution of management and results. *Dis. Colon. Rectum.* **1999**, *42*, 460–466; discussion 466–469. [CrossRef]
29. Agachan, F.; Reissman, P.; Pfeifer, J.; Weiss, E.G.; Nogueras, J.J.; Wexner, S.D. Comparison of three perineal procedures for the treatment of rectal prolapse. *South. Med. J.* **1997**, *90*, 925–932. [CrossRef]
30. Boccasanta, P.; Venturi, M.; Agradi, S.; Calabrò, G.; Bordoni, L.; Missaglia, C.; Favetta, U.; Vergani, C. Is it possible to reduce recurrences after Altemeier's procedure for complete rectal prolapse? Twenty-year experience in 130 consecutive patients. *Langenbecks Arch. Surg.* **2021**, *406*, 1591–1598. [CrossRef]
31. Takesue, Y.; Yokoyama, T.; Murakami, Y.; Akagi, S.; Ohge, H.; Yokoyama, Y.; Sakashita, Y.; Tatsumoto, N.; Miyamoto, K.; Matsuura, Y. The effectiveness of perineal rectosigmoidectomy for the treatment of rectal prolapse in elderly and high-risk patients. *Surg. Today* **1999**, *29*, 290–293. [CrossRef]
32. Lee, S.H.; Lakhtaria, P.; Canedo, J.; Lee, Y.S.; Wexner, S.D. Outcome of laparoscopic rectopexy versus perineal rectosigmoidectomy for full-thickness rectal prolapse in elderly patients. *Surg. Endosc.* **2011**, *25*, 2699–2702. [CrossRef] [PubMed]
33. Senapati, A.; Gray, R.G.; Middleton, L.J.; Harding, J.; Hills, R.K.; Armitage, N.C.; Buckley, L.; Northover, J.M.; PROSPER Collaborative Group. PROSPER: A randomised comparison of surgical treatments for rectal prolapse. *Color. Dis.* **2013**, *15*, 858–868. [CrossRef] [PubMed]
34. Marzouk, D.; Ramdass, M.J.; Haji, A.; Akhtar, M. Digital assessment of lower rectum fixity in rectal prolapse (DALR): A simple clinical anatomical test to determine the most suitable approach (abdominal versus perineal) for repair. *Surg. Radiol. Anat.* **2005**, *27*, 414–419. [CrossRef]
35. Nguyen, X.H.; Pham, P.K.; Steinhagen, R.M.; Pham, G.A.; Le, N.H.; Nguyen, N.A. Case series: Incarcerated massive rectal prolapse successfully treated with Altemeier's procedure. *Int. J. Surg. Case Rep.* **2018**, *51*, 309–312. [CrossRef] [PubMed]
36. De Schlichting, T.; Poncet, G.; Bufacchi, P.; Pasquer, A. An emergency Altemeier procedure for necrosis of full-thickness rectal prolapse. *Tech. Coloproctol.* **2021**, *25*, 1165. [CrossRef]
37. Pandit, N.; Yadav, T.N.; Awale, L. Incarcerated complete rectal prolapse managed by Altemeier's procedure. *Trop. Doct.* **2020**, *50*, 236–238. [CrossRef]
38. Koizumi, N.; Kobayashi, H.; Fukumoto, K. Massive chronic irreducible rectal prolapse successfully treated with Altemeier's procedure. *J. Surg. Case Rep.* **2018**, *2018*, rjy064. [CrossRef] [PubMed]
39. Johansen, O.B.; Wexner, S.D.; Daniel, N.; Nogueras, J.J.; Jagelman, D.G. Perineal rectosigmoidectomy in the elderly. *Dis. Colon. Rectum.* **1993**, *36*, 767–772. [CrossRef] [PubMed]
40. Ramanujam, P.S.; Venkatesh, K.S.; Fietz, M.J. Perineal excision of rectal procidentia in elderly high-risk patients. A ten-year experience. *Dis. Colon. Rectum.* **1994**, *37*, 1027–1030. [CrossRef]
41. Deen, K.I.; Grant, E.; Billingham, C.; Keighley, M.R. Abdominal resection rectopexy with pelvic floor repair versus perineal rectosigmoidectomy and pelvic floor repair for full-thickness rectal prolapse. *Br. J. Surg.* **1994**, *81*, 302–304. [CrossRef] [PubMed]
42. Zbar, A.P.; Takashima, S.; Hasegawa, T.; Kitabayashi, K. Perineal rectosigmoidectomy (Altemeier's procedure): A review of physiology, technique and outcome. *Tech. Coloproctol.* **2002**, *6*, 109–116. [CrossRef]
43. Habr-Gama, A.; Jacob, C.E.; Jorge, J.M.; Seid, V.E.; Marques, C.F.; Mantese, J.C.; Kiss, D.R.; Gama-Rodrigues, J. Rectal procidentia treatment by perineal rectosigmoidectomy combined with levator ani repair. *Hepatogastroenterology* **2006**, *53*, 213–217.

44. Boccasanta, P.; Venturi, M.; Barbieri, S.; Roviaro, G. Impact of new technologies on the clinical and functional outcome of Altemeier's procedure: A randomized, controlled trial. *Dis. Colon. Rectum.* **2006**, *49*, 652–660. [CrossRef] [PubMed]
45. Trompetto, M.; Tutino, R.; Realis Luc, A.; Novelli, E.; Gallo, G.; Clerico, G. Altemeier's procedure for complete rectal prolapse; outcome and function in 43 consecutive female patients. *BMC Surg.* **2019**, *19*, 1. [CrossRef] [PubMed]

Journal of *Personalized Medicine*

MDPI

Review

Knockout Genes in Bowel Anastomoses: A Systematic Review of Literature Outcomes

Georgios Geropoulos [1,†], Kyriakos Psarras [1,*,†], Georgios Koimtzis [1], Massimiliano Fornasiero [2], Elissavet Anestiadou [3], Vasileios Geropoulos [1], Anna Michopoulou [1,4], Maria Papaioannou [4], Kokkona Kouzi-Koliakou [5] and Ioannis Galanis [1]

1 2nd Department of Propaedeutic Surgery, Hippokration Hospital, School of Medicine, Aristotle University of Thessaloniki, 54642 Thessaloniki, Greece; georgios.geropoulos@nhs.net (G.G.); drgxkoimtzis@gmail.com (G.K.); geropoulosv@gmail.com (V.G.); annamichop@yahoo.gr (A.M.); galanis@auth.gr (I.G.)

2 Medical School, University College London, London WC1E6DE, UK; maxfornasiero@googlemail.com

3 Fourth Surgical Department, School of Medicine, Aristotle University of Thessaloniki, 57010 Thessaloniki, Greece; elissavetxatz@gmail.com

4 Laboratory of Biological Chemistry, School of Medicine, Aristotle University of Thessaloniki, 54124 Thessaloniki, Greece; mpapaioannou@auth.gr

5 Laboratory of Histology and Embryology, Medical School, Aristotle University of Thessaloniki, 54124 Thessaloniki, Greece; kkoliako@auth.gr

* Correspondence: psarrask@auth.gr

† These authors contributed equally to this work.

Abstract: Background: The intestinal wound healing process is a complex event of three overlapping phases: exudative, proliferative, and remodeling. Although some mechanisms have been extensively described, the intestinal healing process is still not fully understood. There are some similarities but also some differences compared to other tissues. The aim of this systematic review was to summarize all studies with knockout (KO) experimental models in bowel anastomoses, underline any recent knowledge, and clarify further the cellular and molecular mechanisms of the intestinal healing process. A systematic review protocol was performed. Materials and methods: Medline, EMBASE, and Scopus were comprehensively searched. Results: a total of eight studies were included. The silenced genes included interleukin-10, the four-and-one-half LIM domain-containing protein 2 (FHL2), cyclooxygenase-2 (COX-2), annexin A1 (ANXA-1), thrombin-activatable fibrinolysis inhibitor (TAFI), and heparin-binding epidermal growth factor (HB-EGF) gene. Surgically, an end-to-end bowel anastomosis was performed in the majority of the studies. Increased inflammatory cell infiltration in the anastomotic site was found in IL-10-, annexin-A1-, and TAFI-deficient mice compared to controls. COX-1 deficiency showed decreased angiogenesis at the anastomotic site. Administration of prostaglandin E2 in COX-2-deficient mice partially improved anastomotic leak rates, while treatment of ANXA1 KO mice with Ac2-26 nanoparticles reduced colitis activity and increased weight recovery following surgery. Conclusions: our findings provide new insights into improving intestinal wound healing by amplifying the aforementioned genes using appropriate gene therapies. Further research is required to clarify further the cellular and micromolecular mechanisms of intestinal healing.

Keywords: knockout genes; anastomosis; rat; surgery; intestinal wound healing

1. Introduction

Anastomosis construction is considered one of the most crucial steps in gastrointestinal (GI) surgery. An anastomotic leak is a potentially fatal complication, resulting in higher reoperation rates as well worse prognosis, with increased morbidity and mortality [1–3]. Furthermore, apart from the physical and psychological burden, an anastomotic leak represents a significant economic burden for healthcare facilities, mainly due to prolonged hospital stay [4]. Despite progress in GI surgery techniques and materials, GI anastomoses currently present high leakage rates; up to 4% for ileocolic, 18% for colorectal, and 19% for coloanal anastomoses [5]. The problem is exacerbated in patients with inflammatory diseases, sepsis, malnutrition, or in those receiving steroids, immunosuppressives, and neoadjuvant radio-chemotherapy [6].

There are three phases of intestinal wound healing, including inflammation, proliferation, and remodeling, which partly occur simultaneously. The inflammatory phase begins immediately after injury, in which leukocytes infiltrate the submucosa along with accompanying oedema. This process lasts for two weeks, initially with a neutrophil-rich acute response which slowly changes into a chronic macrophage response. Fibroblast and smooth muscle cell proliferation lead to small amounts of collagen formation in order to initially strengthen the anastomosis. Mucosal resurfacing starts early and is completed within one week. Remodeling starts after one week through additional collagen formation and substitution of the already existing collagen with stronger types of collagen. However, the architecture of muscularis mucosa and muscularis propria remains irregular compared to healthy tissue [7].

Intestinal anastomosis healing follows a process quite similar to that encountered in other tissues, with some remarkable differences. The rate of healing in the GI tract is rapid (weeks), whereas in the skin it is more prolonged (months) [8]. The serosa in the GI tract give additional healing strength. The shear stress in the GI tract is increased due to intraluminal bulk transit and peristalsis. GI healing bears a high aerobic and anaerobic bacterial load while skin only has aerobic bacteria. A study from Wahl et al. showed that E. coli species' predomination in the GI tract can produce toxins, disrupting epithelial integrity and collagen synthesis [9]. Another difference exists in the cellular source of collagen; fibroblasts are responsible for this in the skin, whereas smooth muscle cells are responsible for this in the GI tissues [10]. Furthermore, there are differences in the healing process between different sections of the GI tract. For example, collagen synthesis occurs more rapidly in the ileum compared to the colon [8]. Small bowel anastomosis strength approaches the strength of unwounded tissue about four weeks post injury, while the large bowel needs four months to gain only 75% of its initial strength.

Despite our knowledge of GI healing processes, there are still many molecules and molecule interactions to be identified in order to get a complete idea of their importance and their participation in serious complications, such as improper healing leading to anastomotic leak. A useful tool to explore and analyze the action of certain molecules is the use of knockout mice. Knockout (KO) mice are genetically modified laboratory animals lacking a certain gene and its codified protein. KO mice have been increasingly utilized in recent years to study the immunological and molecular mechanisms involved in anastomotic would healing and interactions therein. This systematic review aims to summarize all significant findings of KO mice experiments in GI wound healing and potentially clarify their relationship to anastomotic leak occurrence.

2. Materials and Methods

2.1. Study Design and Inclusion/Exclusion Criteria

This systematic review was conducted according to the Preferred Reporting Items for Systematic Reviews and Meta-Analyses (PRISMA) guidelines, in line with the protocol developed and agreed a priori by all authors. Studies investigating the impact of genetic KO mouse or rat models' effects on bowel anastomosis integrity were deemed eligible for analysis. Control mice or rats among the studies were animals that received no intervention, drinking normal water, or being mentioned in the text as wild-type animals. Exclusion criteria were as follows: (i) articles published in languages other than English, (ii) narrative or systematic reviews and meta-analyses, (iii) case reports, errata, comments, perspectives, letters to the editor, and editorials that did not provide any extractable data, (iv) published abstracts with no available full text, and (v) non-comparative studies (single-arm studies). No publication date, sample size restrictions, or any other search filters were applied.

2.2. Search Strategy

Eligible studies were identified by searching through the MEDLINE (via PubMed), Cochrane Library, Embase, and Scopus databases (end-of-search date: 1 October 2023). These searches were conducted by two independent researchers. The search strategies used were the following: (knockout) AND (anastom*). The search algorithm included all of the available synonyms and related terms. Any disagreements were resolved by a third reviewer. The reference lists and all previously published systematic reviews were thoroughly searched for missed studies eligible for inclusion based on the "snowball" methodology [11].

2.3. Data Extraction

A standardized, pre-piloted form was used for data tabulation and extraction. Two reviewers extracted the data independently, and any disagreements were identified and resolved by a third reviewer. We extracted the following data from the included studies: study characteristics (first author, year of publication, country, and number of mice in each group), (ii) gene characteristics (KO gene, gene function, underlying condition), (iii) operation characteristics (method of anastomosis, suture material), and (iv) post-operative analysis (hydroxyproline, bursting pressure, histological characteristics).

3. Results

3.1. Study Characteristics

A total of one hundred and forty studies were identified and a total of eight studies were included for data extraction, published between 2003 and 2021 [12–19]. Two studies were from Germany [15,16], two studies were from the USA [12,13], another two were from the Netherlands [14,18], one was from Canada [19], and one from China [17]. All studies included KO mouse models. A total of 767 mice were included in the review, averaging 95.9 mice per study (Table 1). A flow diagram is shown in Figure 1.

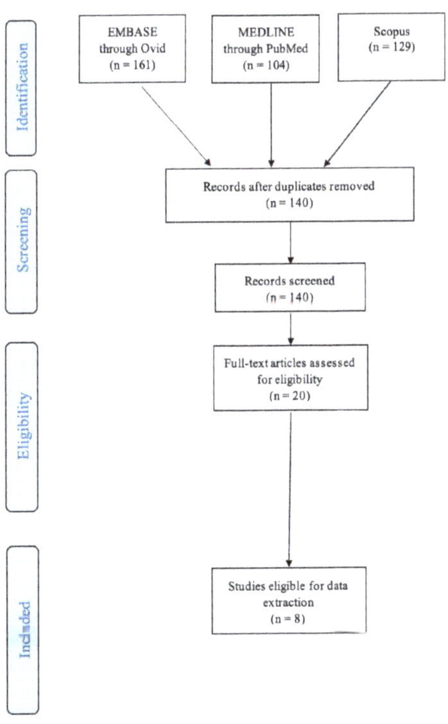

Figure 1. PRISMA flowchart.

Table 1. Summary of the study details and genetic knockout characteristics. ANXA1 = annexin A1, COX-2 = cyclooxygenase-2, HB-EGF = heparin-binding epidermal growth factor, IL-10 = interleukin-10, KO = knockout, MAPK = mitogen-activated protein kinase, NA = not applicable, NSAID = non-steroidal anti-inflammatory drug, SHIP1 = Src homology-2 domain-containing inositol 5-phosphatase 1, TAFI = thrombin-activatable fibrinolysis inhibitor, TG = transgenic, VEGF = vascular endothelial growth factor, WT = wild type (act as control for the genetically altered mice).

Study (Year)	Country	Knockout Gene	Gene Function	Underlying Condition	Groups (Number of Participants, n)
Borowiec et al. (2012) [19]	Canada	IL-10 129/SvEv background (the strain of mice used for experimentation)	IL-10 production	Crohn's disease	Control WT (no intervention) (n = 18) Control IL-10 null (no intervention) (n = 18) Ileocolonic anastomosis WT (n = 18) Ileocolonic anastomosis IL-10 null (n = 18) Sham surgery WT (n = 18) Sham surgery IL-10 null (n = 18)
Wu et al. (2013) [17]	China	miR-155/SHIP-1 pathway, responsible for epigenetic modification, altering transcription rates and cell turnover	Th1/Th2 regulator Increased miR-155 promotes differentiation into CD4+ cells and inhibits CD8+ differentiation	Crohn's disease	IL-10 KO control (no intervention) (n = 6) IL-10 KO ileocecal anastomosis + intraperitoneal saline injection (n = 6) IL-10 KO ileocecal anastomosis + intraperitoneal triptolide injection (n = 6) WT control (no intervention) (n = 6)
Kirfel et al. (2008) [16]	Germany	FHL2	Multifactorial cofactor for gene transcription, negatively regulates MAPK signaling	Crohn's disease	WT (n = 68) FHL2-deficient mice (n = 70)
Rigby et al. (2009) [12]	USA	IL-10 129/SvEv background	IL-10 production	Crohn's disease	WT ileo-cecal resection (n = 10) WT sham (n = 8) WT no surgery (n = 3) IL-10 null ileo-cecal resection (n = 11) IL-10 null sham (n = 5) IL-10 null no surgery (n = 6)
Reisinger et al. (2017) [14]	The Netherlands	COX-2	Immune modulation, myofibroblast proliferation, VEGF-induced angiogenesis through prostaglandin production	NA—mimic NSAID use	WT (n = 32) COX-2 + / − (n = 17) COX-2 KO (n = 25)

Table 1. *Cont.*

Study (Year)	Country	Knockout Gene	Gene Function	Underlying Condition	Groups (Number of Participants, *n*)
Reischl et al. (2021) [15]	Germany	ANXA1	Annexin A1 generation—anti-inflammatory protein inhibiting leukocyte activation and transmigration	Colitis	WT-induced colitis (n = 36) Anxa1-KO-induced colitis (n = 36) Colitis + anastomosis (n = 56) Control (normal drinking water without DSS) + anastomosis (n = 36) Colitis + anastomosis + Ac2-26-nanoparticles (n = 24) Colitis + anastomosis + sham Ac2-26-nanoparticles (n = 24)
Te Velde et al. (2003) [13]	The Netherlands	TAFI	Downregulates fibrinolysis	NA	WT mice (n = 14) TAFI knockout mice (n = 14)
Radulescu et al. (2011) [[illegible]3]	USA	HB-EGF	Mitogen, chemoattractant for smooth muscle cells and fibroblasts	NA	HB-EGF KO (n = 42) HB-EGF +/+ WT (n = 33) HB-EGF TG mice (n = 26) WT (n = 27) WT mice with enteral HB-EGF added (n = 21)

3.2. *Experimental Animals Characteristics*

Three studies used IL-10 KO mice [12,17,19]. In one of these studies, triptolide was used to reverse the pro-inflammatory effect of IL-10 deficiency [17]. These mice subsequently developed Crohn's disease as a result of IL-10 deficiency. One study modeled Crohn's disease by FHL2 deletion, a multifactorial cofactor for gene transcription which negatively regulates mitogen-activated protein kinase (MAPK) signaling [16]. Another study used cyclooxygenase-2 (COX-2) KO mice mimicking a non-steroidal anti-inflammatory drug (NSAID) effect. The result was immune modulation, myoblast proliferation, and reduced vascular-endothelial-growth-factor- (VEGF-) induced angiogenesis [14]. One study used annexin A1 (Anxa1) gene KO mice to induce inflammatory colitis by leukocyte activation and transmigration [15]. Another study used thrombin-activatable fibrinolysis inhibitor (TAFI) KO mice, compared to wild type (WT) mouse models, for anastomotic studies [18]. One study used heparin-binding epidermal growth factor (HB-EGF) KO mice for their experiments, again compared to WT mice used as control [13] (Table 1).

3.3. *Operative Characteristics*

The majority of studies used interrupted sutures to form an end-to-end anastomosis [12–17]. One study used continuous sutures for their end-to-end anastomosis [18] and another study formed a side-to-side anastomosis with interrupted sutures [19]. Three studies used 8-0 prolene for the anastomosis [14,18,19]. Two used 9-0 nylon [12,17], and one used 4-0 nylon [13]. Two studies used vicryl sutures [15,16] (Table 2).

Table 2. Summary of operative details, histological and inflammatory analysis, and bursting pressure. ANXA1 = annexin A1, COX-2 = cyclooxygenase-2, HB-EGF = heparin-binding epidermal growth factor, IL-10 = interleukin-10, KO = knockout, MMP = matrix metalloproteinase, NA = not assessed, POD = postoperative day, TAFI = thrombin-activatable fibrinolysis inhibitor, TG = transgenic, VEGF = vascular endothelial growth factor, WT = wild type.

Study (Year)	Method of Anastomosis	Suture Material	Histology	Bursting Pressure	Inflammatory Effect
Borowiec et al. (2012) [19]	Interrupted sutures, side-to-side anastomosis	8-0 Prolene	No collagen difference between WT and IL-10 null mice	NA	Increased lymphocyte infiltration in IL-10 KO
Wu et al. (2013) [17]	Interrupted sutures, end-to-end anastomosis	9-0 nylon	Epithelial cell hyperplasia, mucin depletion, and crypt abscess formation in anastomosis group, reversed by administration of triptolide	NA	Increased lymphocytic infiltration in anastomosis group compared to control, reversed by administration of triptolide
Kirfel et al. (2008) [16]	Interrupted sutures, end-to-end anastomosis	8-0 polyglactin	Reduced submucosal collagen type I and III deposition in FHL-2-deficient mice around injury site, no difference in unaffected bowel compared to control	Lower bursting pressure in FHL-2-deficient mice at days 2, 5, and 14 postoperatively	NA
Rigby et al. (2009) [12]	Interrupted sutures, end-to-end anastomosis	9-0 nylon	Increased collagen mRNA in small intestine of IL-10 null mice compared to WT Reduced fibrosis in germ-free IL-10 null mice compared to conventional IL-10 null mice	NA	Inflammation in IL-10 null mice after ileo-cecal resection in the small intestine and anastomosis No difference between WT mice of different treatment groups
Reisinger et al. (2017) [14]	Interrupted sutures, end-to-end anastomosis	8-0 Prolene	Significantly reduced vascularization, reduced VEGF levels in COX-2 KO compared to WT	NA	No inflammatory differences observed between WT and COX-2 KO
Reischl et al. (2021) [15]	Interrupted sutures, end-to-end anastomosis	9-0 Vicryl	Increased MMP expression on POD1 in ANXA1 KO compared to WT mice Ac2-26 nanoparticles improved histological healing scores compared to control	Healthy mice	Higher inflammation score in Anxa1 KO mice compared with WT Ac2-26 nanoparticles reduced colitis activity and suppressed pro-inflammatory cytokine expression
Te Velde et al. (2003) [18]	Continuous sutures, end-to-end anastomosis	8-0 Prolene	POD7: no gross differences in granulation tissue between KO and WT mice	Significantly lower in TAFI KO compared to WT Burst on anastomosis line in 4/14 TAFI KO mice, but normal intestinal tissue in all WT mice	Increased inflammation only in 4/14 TAFI KO mice following anastomotic leak
Radulescu et al. (2011) [13]	Interrupted sutures, end-to-end anastomosis	4-0 Nylon	KO mice demonstrated worse healing scores compared to WT, which were worse than HB-EGF TG Increased collagen deposition and increased mature vascularization of anastomosis in TG mice compared to KO mice	HB-EGF KO < WT < HB-EGF TG	KO mice demonstrated increased inflammation compared to WT, which was increased compared to HB-EGF TG

3.4. Histological Characteristics

All studies assessed the histological characteristics of the bowel anastomosis in gene KO mice. In IL-10 KO mice, a study found no significant difference in collagen deposition between IL-10 KO mice and control [19], while another study found significantly increased collagen mRNA in IL-10 KO mice compared to WT mice. This additional collagen mRNA translated into increased collagen deposition and fibrosis at the anastomosis [12]. The microbiome is also likely to play a role, with reduced fibrosis in germ-free IL-10 KO mice compared to conventional IL-10 KO mice [12], although the exact mechanisms have not been identified. Wu et al. [17] found epithelial cell hyperplasia, mucin depletion, and crypt abscess formation in IL-10 deficient mice at the anastomosis site and more extensively throughout the bowel.

FHL2 KO mice demonstrated reduced submucosal collagen type I and III deposition around the injury site, with no difference in collagen in areas of unaffected bowel compared to WT mice acting as controls [16]. Inhibition of COX-2 correlated with reduced vascularization around the anastomosis site compared to controls [14]. Annexin A1 KO mice demonstrated a reduced histological healing score (Scored 0–4 for inflammatory cells, angiogenesis, collagen synthesis, fibroblast ingrowth, and overall healing quality, adapted from Phillips et al. [20]) compared to control, which was improved with the addition of Ac2-26 nanoparticles [15]. TAFI KO mice showed no differences in granulation tissue deposition between the KO group and WT [18]. HB-EGF KO mice showed reduced healing scores compared to WT. Transgenic (TG) HB-EGF mice, engineered to overexpress HB-EGF resulting in additional HB-EGF produced, showed increased collagen deposition and mature vascularization around the anastomosis site compared to WT mice [13]. Seven studies assessed inflammation differences around the anastomosis site [12–15,17–19]. IL-10 KO mouse models showed increased lymphocyte infiltration when compared to WT mice that faced either surgical intervention or a non-operative study arm [12,17,19]. This was reversed with administration of triptolide [17]. Increased inflammation (defined as increased numbers of morphonuclear leukocytes, lymphocytes, and macrophages on histological analysis) was found in HB-EGF KO, compared to WT, which demonstrated increased inflammation compared to TG HB-EGD mice [13]. Increased inflammation and matrix metalloproteinase (MMP) expression was found in Anxa1 KO mice compared to WT, with reduced inflammation upon addition of Ac2-26 nanoparticles [15]. However, no anastomotic area inflammatory differences were noted between COX-2 KO mice and WT mice [14]. Interestingly, Te Velde et al. [18] only found increased inflammation around the anastomotic site in TAFI KO mice who experienced anastomotic leak, but not in other TAFI KO mice (Table 2).

3.5. Bursting Pressure

Three studies assessed bursting pressure. Kirfel et al. [16] demonstrated a reduced bursting pressure in FHL2 KO mice compared to control at days 2, 5, and 14, postoperatively. TAFI KO mice also had a reduced bursting pressure despite no granulation tissue differences when compared to WT mice [18]. HB-EDF KO mice had reduced bursting pressure compared to WT mice. TG HB-EGF mice had increased bursting pressure when compared to WT, again correlating with collagen deposition noted on histological analysis [13] (Table 2).

4. Discussion

Bowel resection and anastomosis represents a significant component of GI disease surgical management. Anastomotic leak represents a severe post-operative complication, with varying incidence up to 36% [21]. The clinical presentation of leaks varies significantly, from low-grade fever and overall delayed recovery of the patient to severe peritonitis and sepsis [22]. This results in longer inpatient stays, increased mortality, and higher healthcare expenses [23–25]. Therefore, it is of utmost importance to elucidate intestinal wound healing pathways in order to find ways to improve healing and reduce the incidence of anastomotic leaks. This systematic review identified several studies investigating the lack of the following molecules: IL-10, cyclooxygenase-2, annexin A1, TAFI, and heparin-binding epidermal growth factor genes. Increased inflammatory cell infiltration in the anastomotic site was found in IL-10-, annexin-A1-, and TAFI-deficient mice compared to controls. COX-1 deficiency showed decreased angiogenesis at the anastomotic site. Our findings provide new ways to improve intestinal wound healing through amplifying the aforementioned genes with appropriate gene therapies. Genetic modification of mouse models has translated into different results of clinical parameters. Various agents have been shown to be useful in reducing anastomotic leaks and their relative complications. For example, Radulescu et al. [13] generated mouse models over-expressing HB-EGF. This increased bursting pressure and collagen deposition. In a different included study conducted by Reischl et al., Ac2-26 nanoparticles added to ANXA1 KO mice improved histological healing [15]. Addition of prostaglandin E2 in COX-2-deficient mice partially improved anastomotic leak rates, closer to those of WT mice [14]. HB-EGF KO mice models led to higher mortality and complication rates (including bleeding, anastomotic dehiscence, abscess formation, and obstruction) [13]. Treatment of ANXA1 KO mice with Ac2-26 nanoparticles reduced colitis activity and increased weight recovery following surgery [15]. Use of diclofenac to inhibit COX-2 resulted in significantly increased rates of anastomotic leak compared to control [14]. TAFI KO mice had significantly increased weight loss, adhesions, bleeding, and mortality compared to WT mice [18].

4.1. Interleukin 10, miR-155/SHIP-1 Pathway and Wound Healing

IL-10, as a regulatory cytokine of inflammation, has been the subject of extensive study in the context of anastomotic healing. IL-10 is primarily produced from macrophages residing in the lamina propria of the bowel and regulatory T-cells in order to reduce the immune response to proinflammatory molecules on cell membranes of local bacteria [26]. In addition, epithelial cells and Th1 cells triggered by lipoproteins of commensal bacteria are capable of producing IL-10 in order to maintain bowel homeostasis [27,28]. Incubation of IL-10 KO mice's intestinal epithelial cells with recombinant IL-10 enhanced wound repair in vitro because IL-10 binding reversed the KO effect [29]. In vivo, macrophage-derived IL-10 was crucial for small intestine epithelial healing during the acute phase of injury, ultimately driving re-epithelialization in the small intestine [30]. The exact mechanism through which IL-10 promotes bowel wound healing remains unclear. Following biopsy-induced injury, IL-10 activates cyclic adenosine monophosphate (c-AMP) Response-Element-Binding Protein (CREB) signaling and its downstream target WNT1-inducible-signaling pathway protein 1 (WISP-1). This, in turn, promotes β-catenin signaling to induce epithelial proliferation and wound closure [31]. It is therefore possible that IL-10 works directly on epithelial cells. An alternative mechanism suggests that IL-10 works primarily on immune cells, resulting indirectly in wound healing. IL-10 binding to CD11b myeloid cells regulates T cell activation and proliferation of intestinal crypt cells [12,32]. The broad functions of IL-10 have generated significant interest in it as a therapeutic target for multiple disease states. Significant research involving manipulation of IL-10 has been undertaken in the context of inflammatory bowel disease (IBD) [25]. IL-10-deficient mice develop colitis [33], which is managed successfully following administration of IL-10 [34,35]. In 1993, Kühn et al. [36] showed that interleukin-10-deficient (IL-10−/−) mice presented a Th1-mediated chronic colitis similar to human IBD. However, administration of recombinant IL-10 yielded only a minor clinical improvement in the treatment of IBD in humans [37], likely due to the low concentrations achieved in the gut following systemic administration. Lactococcus lactis bacteria, modified to deliver IL-10 to the gut, improved clinical disease scores of a small number of Crohn's disease patients [38]. The effects of IL-10 have also been studied in dermal wound healing. Fetal skin has a tendency to regenerate, whereas postnatal skin heals with scar formation. Fetal skin has elevated levels of IL-10, promoting high molecular weight hyaluronan formation, which reduces inflammation and fibrosis [39,40]. IL-10 administration in IL-10-deficient mice resulted in reduced inflammatory cell numbers and restoration of normal skin architecture, with reduced scar size. This resulted in accelerated dermal healing and increased tissue strength [41]. Regarding IBD, it has been demonstrated that triptolide ameliorates the severity of IL-10-deficient mouse colitis via inhibition of TLRs (toll-like receptors)/NF-κB and IL-6/STAT3 signaling pathways, and down-regulation of IL-17 [42,43]. Triptolide is a bioactive compound produced by the plant Tripterygium wilfordii Hook F (TwHF) and has been widely used in clinical practice due to its anti-inflammatory and immunosuppressive properties [44]. Its mechanisms of action include the following: (1) inhibition of expression of RPB1 (the RNA polymerase II main subunit), (2) inhibition of xeroderma pigmentosum group B (XPB) protein, which is a subunit of transcription factor II-H, and (3) inhibition of induction of miR-155 in LPS-stimulated macrophages [17]. In particular, miR-155 targets SHIP-1 (Src-homology-2-containing inositol phosphatase-1), which is an inhibitor of many inflammatory processes and regulates the balance of T cell subsets [17,42,43].

4.2. *Cyclooxygenase (COX) and Wound Healing*

COX is an essential enzyme in the synthesis of prostaglandins, occurring in two isoforms. COX1 is constitutively expressed, whereas COX2 is expressed in response to injury. In dermal injury, COX-2 expression peaks 3 days later, when the anastomosis is thinnest and at increased risk of rupture [45]. The quantity of COX-2 produced also correlates with the magnitude of the inflammatory response [46]. Hypoxia, partly due to connective tissue deposition during wound healing, stimulates angiogenesis through HIF-1α induction of VEGF secretion. VEGF is also responsible for fibroblast differentiation and tissue remodeling. The COX–VEGF axis plays an important role in wound healing, since pharmacologically induced downregulation of COX-2 correlates with significantly increased VEGF levels. A study of full-thickness skin incisions in mice demonstrated increased angiogenesis and collagen deposition on histology, which correlated with a significant increase in wound contraction and reduced wound area macroscopically [47]. These findings are in contrast to those of another paper included in our analysis, indicating that COX-2 KO mice demonstrate reduced VEGF-induced angiogenesis at the anastomosis [14]. This could be due to an alternative mechanism for VEGF production, or a difference in healing between dermal and bowel injury. However, COX-2 and the resulting production of prostaglandin E2 have been shown to accelerate healing of gastric ulcers, further demonstrating the importance of this pathway in gastrointestinal mucosal repair [48]. Prostaglandin (PG) biosynthesis is mediated by the synergic action of two enzymes: phospholipase, responsible for the metabolism of arachidonic acid (AA) from cell membrane phospholipids, and COX. Prostaglandin E2 (PGE2) is the most abundant and important COX-2 product regarding intestinal wound healing [49]. Under normal conditions, the PGE2 signaling pathway can potentially trigger stem cell differentiation towards enterocytes [50]. After an injury, epithelial restitution is a crucial process that is performed in the intestine by a special cell population with transient repair features named wound-associated epithelial cells (WAE) and, in combination with non-canonical Wnt signaling activation, this ensures controlled wound repair [51]. Epithelial restitution is a protective mechanism including the migration of epithelial cells from intact wound margin into the injured basal lamina to reseal the intestinal barrier. Miyoshi et al. showed that PGE2 signaling through its receptor promotes WAE differentiation of intestinal epithelial stem cells in an in vitro model. In vivo studies in mice with depletion of the PGE2 receptor led to insufficient intestinal wound repair due to impaired production of WAE cells, and they exhibited impaired wound repair [52]. In addition, it has been found that increased COX-2 expression is noted in macrophages and myofibroblasts after exposure to proinflammatory signals, triggering intestinal tissue proliferation [14]. Numerous studies have shown the regenerative role of PGE2, a product of the COX-2 gene, for intestinal wall repair under a wide range of pathological circumstances, such as dextran-sulfate-sodium- (DSS-) induced inflammation and ischemia-reperfusion injury [53,54]. In addition, PGE2 and COX-2, through activation of the PGE2 receptor and following upregulation of VEGF expression, stimulate neoangiogenesis but also promote the proliferation and migration of epithelial intestinal cells [55]. Finally, PGE2 regulates myofibroblast function, which is responsible for producing collagen, the main structural component of the extracellular matrix [56]. In terms of clinical application, there is conflicting evidence regarding whether COX-2 blockage is associated with impaiastomotic leak development. Two recent meta-analyses involving patients undergoing operations for colorectal cancer have concluded in undetermined relationships between postoperative NSAID administration and anastomotic leakage [57,58]. On the other hand, a subgroup analysis by Jamjittrong et al. focused on colorectal anastomoses revealed a significantly increased anastomotic leakage rate in patients who were administered NSAIDs perioperatively [57]. In human genome studies, the PTGS2 −765G > C polymorphism lies in the promoter region of the gene that encodes COX-2 and leads to lower levels of COX-2 [59]. Reisinger and Makar suggested that the homozygous state for PTGS2-765G > C polymorphism, which is encountered with a prevalence of 3% in humans, led to decreased COX-2 expression and increased anastomotic leakage rates [14,60].

4.3. Anxa1 and Wound Healing

Annexin A1 (AnxA1), also named lipocortin-1, is a calcium-dependent phospholipid-binding protein from the family of SPMs. Clinical studies have shown that higher AnxA1 expression is associated with milder symptomatology and severity in both Crohn's disease (CD) and ulcerative colitis (UC) [61]. A 26-amino acid ANXA1 N-terminal peptide Ac2-26, a part of the full-length molecule, is the active part of ANXA1 [62]. AnxA1's anti-inflammatory role is based on inhibition of neutrophil accumulation, transendothelial migration, and activation, as well as promotion of neutrophil apoptosis after binding to the formyl peptide receptor 2 (FPR2/ALX) and formyl peptide receptor 1 (FPR1) [15]. In addition, AnxA1 induces monocyte chemotaxis and removal of apoptotic leukocytes by macrophages. It promotes keratinocytes' motility and differentiation, which is important for wound re-epithelization [63]. Finally, AnxA1 controls macrophage cell reprogramming towards reduced production of proinflammatory molecules and increased production of anti-inflammatory agents [64]. Annexin 2 is a calcium-dependent phospholipid-binding protein associated with cytoskeleton coordination [65]. Through annexin 2 [66], epithelial cell migration re-establishes the epithelial barrier and reseals the mucosal defect of the bowel following surgery. Our review included a study [15] investigating the role of annexin A1 on the resolution of inflammation following surgery for colitis. Epithelial injury of the bowel brings into contact the immune cells of the intestinal wall and the lumen's bacteria, resulting in an inflammatory response. Anxa1 is a component of the extracellular vesicles of these immune cells [67]. When released into the extracellular space, it modifies the inflammatory response of phagocytes and epithelial cells through binding to formyl peptide receptors [68]. Our included study [15] found an increased inflammatory score and increased MMP in Anxa1 KO mice, which is consistent with the process described above. Therefore, Anxa1 deficiency reduces epithelial integrity by exposing inflammatory cells to the gut microbiome. Clinically, increased Anxa1 expression in mouse models of CD correlated with histological recovery of the gut mucosa [69]. Further evidence suggests that Anxa1 mediates the positive response of infliximab in CD patients [70].

4.4. FHL2 and Wound Healing

FHL2 belongs to the LIM protein superfamily and exhibits a key role in a wide range of cell functions, including regulation of cell proliferation, gene expression, survival, control of cell architecture, cell adhesion, apoptosis, cell motility, and signal transduction [71]. FHL2 has a distinctive signaling role for mesenchymal cells, controlling their migration, contraction, and differentiation into myofibroblasts through expression of α-smooth muscle actin [16]. During the inflammation phase, FHL2 contributes to pathogen clearance, synthesis, and release of proinflammatory cytokines and immune cell infiltration. During the migration/proliferation phase it has a key role in the function of myofibroblasts, in their differentiation from fibroblasts or from epithelial cells via epithelial mesenchymal transition, and in suppression of MMPs, leading to sufficient contraction and formation of granulation tissue. Finally, during the remodeling phase of the wound healing, FHL2 participates actively in ECM synthesis and remodeling [72]. The literature contains many reports regarding the role of FHL2 in cardiovascular disorders and carcinogenesis [73,74]. However, emerging evidence indicates its role in all phases of wound healing and inflammation. Although under normal conditions FHL2 expression is very low in most tissues, it is upregulated in the skin during wound repair, especially in phases of migration and proliferation. FHL2 suppression is associated with healing failure or prolonged wound healing [72]. In terms of anastomosis healing, Kirfel et al. [16] explored the healing of an end-to-end small bowel anastomosis in FHL2-deficient mice compared to WT mice. They found that FHL2 KO mice presented a statistically significant increase in anastomotic failure rate and lower anastomotic bursting pressure. Histopathologically, insufficient wound healing was noted in anastomotic specimens derived from KO mice, characterized by decreased mucosal and muscular continuity and reduced granulation tissue formation at the fifth and fourteenth postoperative day. On the fifth postoperative day, WT mice presented a dense pattern of organized collagen formation, mainly in the submucosal layer of injured tissue, while submucosa in the FHL2 KO mice presented significantly thinner collagen I/collagen III networks. This was due to downregulation of collagen III mRNA expression in FHL2 KO mice at the anastomotic site. Depletion of FHL2 did not lead to difference in local MMP expression [16].

4.5. HB-EGF and Wound Healing

HB-EGF belongs to the epidermal growth factor (EGF) family. It binds to heparin, as well as to human epidermal growth factor receptors ErbB-1 and ErbB-4, and triggers cellular proliferation, migration, adhesion, and differentiation [75]. Especially for intestinal tissue, it has been shown that HB-EGF exerts a protective effect on intestinal epithelial cells, intestinal stem cells, immunocytes, vascular endothelial cells, pericytes, and intestinal neuronal cells after injury by preserving their cytoskeletal structure and proliferative potential [76,77]. Furthermore, its role in intestinal injury has been delineated in experimental models of necrotizing enterocolitis [78], ischemia/reperfusion injury [79], and resuscitation after hemorrhagic shock [80]. It has been demonstrated that HB-EGF repairs the intestinal epithelium via a phosphatidylinositol 3-kinase (PI3K) and extracellular signal-regulated kinase (ERK)1/2 pathways [81]. Angiogenesis and capillary formation are the basic mechanisms of action of the HB-EGF molecule, which has been shown both in vitro and in vivo [82]. To investigate the role of HB-EGF in intestinal anastomotic healing, Radulescu et al. [13] studied outcomes after division and re-anastomosis of the terminal ileum in HB-EGF KO mice and HB-EGF transgenic (TG) mice. In addition, an extra group of WT mice receiving per os HB-EGF (800 μg/kg) was also included in the experiment [13]. HB-EGF KO mice showed significantly reduced anastomotic bursting pressure and impaired healing scores on the sixth postoperative day. Moreover, higher mortality and greater complication rates postoperatively were reported in HB-EGF KO mice compared to normal controls. Histopathologically, lower collagen levels, severe inflammation in the submucosal space around the anastomosis, and reduced angiogenesis were noted in KO mice. In contrast, HB-EGF TG mice presented increased anastomotic bursting pressure and higher healing scores on the sixth postoperative day, similar mortality, and lower complication rates postoperatively. Histological examination revealed increased angiogenesis and collagen production, minimal signs of inflammation, improved epithelialization, and significant submucosal healing. Per os administration of HB-EGF showed increased anastomotic bursting pressure and significantly lower complication rates. These findings are supportive of the possible cytoprotective role of HB-EGF for intestinal epithelial cells [83].

5. Conclusions

In conclusion, we have identified numerous genes which play crucial roles in anastomotic healing as evidenced by mouse models. IL-10 plays a role in regulating the immune response to prevent excessive inflammation. FHL-2 gene products and HB-EGF improve the structural integrity of the anastomosis, promoting collagen deposition and reducing the bursting pressure. COX-2 gene products are important for signaling VEGF production, contributing to vascularization of the anastomosis.

Author Contributions: Conceptualization, K.P. and G.G.; methodology, G.K. and M.F.; software, G.G.; validation, E.A., V.G. and A.M.; formal analysis, G.G., E.A. and M.F.; investigation, K.P.; resources, G.G.; data curation, M.F., E.A. and K.K.-K.; writing—original draft preparation, G.G., M.F., G.K. and E.A.; writing—review and editing, K.P.; supervision, K.P., K.K.-K., M.P. and I.G.; project administration, K.P. and I.G. All authors have read and agreed to the published version of the manuscript.

Funding: This research received no external funding.

Institutional Review Board Statement: Not applicable.

Informed Consent Statement: Not applicable.

Data Availability Statement: No new data were created. Data taken from previously published studies have been cited in this article.

Conflicts of Interest: The authors declare no conflicts of interest.

References

1. Gessler, B.; Eriksson, O.; Angenete, E. Diagnosis, treatment, and consequences of anastomotic leakage in colorectal surgery. *Int. J. Color. Dis.* **2017**, *32*, 549–556. [CrossRef]
2. Naragund, A.V.; Prabhu, R.Y.; Hira, P.; Karegar, M.M.; Khuroo, S.F.; Bapat, R.D.; Kantharia, C.; Supe, A.N. Can preoperative computed tomography scan predict the occurrence of a pancreatic anastomotic leak: A prospective study with clinical, radiological and pathological co-relation. *Int. J. Hepatobiliary Pancreat. Dis.* **2016**, *6*, 48–56.
3. Espín, E.; Ciga, M.A.; Pera, M.; Ortiz, H.; Lujan, J.; Fraccalvieri, D.; Biondo, S.; Ciga, M.A.; Espí, A.; Codina, A.; et al. Oncological outcome following anastomotic leak in rectal surgery. *J. Br. Surg.* **2015**, *102*, 416–422. [CrossRef] [PubMed]
4. Flor-Lorente, B.; Noguera-Aguilar, J.F.; Delgado-Rivilla, S.; García-González, J.M.; Rodriguez-Martín, M.; Salinas-Ortega, L.; Casado, M.Á.; Álvarez, M. The economic impact of anastomotic leak after colorectal cancer surgery. *Health Econ. Rev.* **2023**, *13*, 12. [CrossRef] [PubMed]
5. Ellis, C.T.; Maykel, J.A. Defining anastomotic leak and the clinical relevance of leaks. *Clin. Colon. Rectal Surg.* **2021**, *34*, 359–365. [CrossRef] [PubMed]
6. Martignoni, M.E.; Friess, H.; Sell, F.; Ricken, L.; Shrikhande, S.; Kulli, C.; Büchler, M.W. Enteral nutrition prolongs delayed gastric emptying in patients after Whipple resection. *Am. J. Surg.* **2000**, *180*, 18–23. [CrossRef] [PubMed]
7. Witte, M.B.; Barbul, A. Repair of full-thickness bowel injury. *Crit. Care Med.* **2003**, *31*, S538–S546. [CrossRef] [PubMed]
8. Thompson, S.K.; Chang, E.Y.; Jobe, B.A. Clinical review: Healing in gastrointestinal anastomoses, part I. *Microsurg. Off. J. Int. Microsurg. Soc. Eur. Fed. Soc. Microsurg.* **2006**, *26*, 131–136. [CrossRef] [PubMed]
9. Wahl, W.; Hassdenteufel, A.; Hofer, B.; Junginger, T. Temporary colostomies after procedures on the sigmoid colon and rectum: Are they still justified? *Langenbecks Arch. Für Chir.* **1997**, *382*, 149–156.
10. Seifert, W.F.; Verhofstad, A.A.; Wobbes, T.; Lange, W.; Rijken, P.F., Van Der Kogel, A.J.; Hendriks, T. Quantitation of angiogenesis in healing anastomoses of the rat colon. *Exp. Mol. Pathol.* **1997**, *64*, 31–40. [CrossRef]
11. National Heart, Lung, and Blood Institute. "Study Quality Assessment Tools," Quality Assessment of Case Control Studies. Available online: https://www.nhlbi.nih.gov/health-topics/study-quality-assessment-tools (accessed on 31 August 2022).
12. Rigby, R.J. A new animal model of postsurgical bowel inflammation and fibrosis: The effect of commensal microflora. *Gut* **2009**, *58*, 1104–1112. [CrossRef]
13. Radulescu, A.; Zhang, H.Y.; Chen, C.L.; Chen, Y.; Zhou, Y.; Yu, X.; Besner, G.E. Heparin-binding EGF-like growth factor promotes intestinal anastomotic healing. *J. Surg. Res.* **2011**, *171*, 540–550. [CrossRef]
14. Reisinger, K.W.; Schellekens, D.H.; Bosmans, J.W.; Boonen, B.; Hulsewé, K.W.; Sastrowijoto, P.; Derikx, J.P.; Grootjans, J.; Poeze, M. Cyclooxygenase-2 Is Essential for Colorectal Anastomotic Healing. *Ann. Surg.* **2017**, *265*, 547–554. [CrossRef] [PubMed]
15. Reischl, S.; Lee, J.H.; Miltschitzky, J.R.E.; Vieregge, V.; Walter, R.L.; Twardy, V.; Kasajima, A.; Friess, H.; Kamaly, N.; Neumann, P.A. AAc2-26-Nanoparticles Induce Resolution of Intestinal Inflammation and Anastomotic Healing via Inhibition of NF-κB Signaling in a Model of Perioperative Colitis. *Inflamm. Bowel Dis.* **2021**, *27*, 1379–1393. [CrossRef]
16. Kirfel, J.; Pantelis, D.; Kabba, M., Kahl, P.; Röper, A.; Kalff, J.C.; Buettner, R. Impaired intestinal wound healing in Fhl2-deficient mice is due to disturbed collagen metabolism. *Exp. Cell Res.* **2008**, *314*, 3684–3691. [CrossRef] [PubMed]
17. Wu, R.; Li, Y.; Guo, Z.; Gong, J.; Zhu, W.; Li, N.; Li, J. Triptolide ameliorates ileocolonic anastomosis inflammation in IL-10 deficient mice by mechanism involving suppression of miR-155/SHIP-1 signaling pathway. *Mol. Immunol.* **2013**, *56*, 340–346. [CrossRef] [PubMed]

18. Te Velde, E.A.; Wagenaar, G.T.; Reijerkerk, A.; Roose-Girma, M.; Borel Rinkes, I.H.; Voest, E.E.; Bouma, B.N.; Gebbink, M.F.; Meijers, J.C. Impaired healing of cutaneous wounds and colonic anastomoses in mice lacking thrombin-activatable fibrinolysis inhibitor. *J. Thromb. Haemost.* **2003**, *1*, 2087–2096. [CrossRef]
19. Borowiec, A.M.; Sydora, B.C.; Doyle, J.; Churchill, T.A.; Madsen, K.; Fedorak, R.N. Small bowel fibrosis and systemic inflammatory response after ileocolonic anastomosis in IL-10 null mice. *J. Surg. Res.* **2012**, *178*, 147–154. [CrossRef] [PubMed]
20. Phillips, J.D.; Kim, C.S.; Fonkalsrud, E.W.; Zeng, H.; Dindar, H. Effects of chronic corticosteroids and vitamin A on the healing of intestinal anastomoses. *Am. J. Surg.* **1992**, *163*, 71–77. [CrossRef]
21. Caulfield, H.; Hyman, N.H. Anastomotic leak after low anterior resection: A spectrum of clinical entities. *JAMA Surg.* **2013**, *148*, 177–182. [CrossRef]
22. Costedio, M.M.; Hyman, N.H. Outcomes of Colorectal Anastomosis. *Semin. Colon. Rectal Surg.* **2008**, *19*, 37–40. [CrossRef]
23. Branagan, G.; Finnis, D. Prognosis after anastomotic leakage in colorectal surgery. *Dis. Colon. Rectum* **2005**, *48*, 1021–1026. [CrossRef]
24. Bakker, I.S.; Grossmann, I.; Henneman, D.; Havenga, K.; Wiggers, T. Risk factors for anastomotic leakage and leak-related mortality after colonic cancer surgery in a nationwide audit. *Br. J. Surg.* **2014**, *101*, 424–432. [CrossRef] [PubMed]
25. Hammond, J.; Lim, S.; Wan, Y.; Gao, X.; Patkar, A. The burden of gastrointestinal anastomotic leaks: An evaluation of clinical and economic outcomes. *J. Gastrointest. Surg.* **2014**, *18*, 1176–1185. [CrossRef] [PubMed]
26. Ueda, Y.; Kayama, H.; Jeon, S.G.; Kusu, T.; Isaka, Y.; Rakugi, H.; Yamamoto, M.; Takeda, K. Commensal microbiota induce LPS hyporesponsiveness in colonic macrophages via the production of IL-10. *Int. Immunol.* **2010**, *22*, 953–962. [CrossRef] [PubMed]
27. Sun, M.; Wu, W.; Chen, L.; Yang, W.; Huang, X.; Ma, C.; Chen, F.; Xiao, Y.; Zhao, Y.; Ma, C.; et al. Microbiota-derived short-chain fatty acids promote Th1 cell IL-10 production to maintain intestinal homeostasis. *Nat. Commun.* **2018**, *9*, 3555. [CrossRef] [PubMed]
28. Latorre, E.; Layunta, E.; Grasa, L.; Pardo, J.; García, S.; Alcalde, A.I.; Mesonero, J.E. Toll-like receptors 2 and 4 modulate intestinal IL-10 differently in ileum and colon. *United Eur. Gastroenterol. J.* **2018**, *6*, 446–453. [CrossRef] [PubMed]
29. Xue, X.; Falcon, D.M. The Role of Immune Cells and Cytokines in Intestinal Wound Healing. *Int. J. Mol. Sci.* **2019**, *20*, 6097. [CrossRef] [PubMed]
30. Morhardt, T.L.; Hayashi, A.; Ochi, T.; Quirós, M.; Kitamoto, S.; Nagao-Kitamoto, H.; Kuffa, P.; Atarashi, K.; Honda, K.; Kao, J.Y.; et al. IL-10 produced by macrophages regulates epithelial integrity in the small intestine. *Sci. Rep.* **2019**, *9*, 1223. [CrossRef] [PubMed]
31. Kim, K.S.; Hong, S.W.; Han, D.; Yi, J.; Jung, J.; Yang, B.G.; Lee, J.Y.; Lee, M.; Surh, C.D. Dietary antigens limit mucosal immunity by inducing regulatory T cells in the small intestine. *Science* **2016**, *351*, 858–863. [CrossRef]
32. Girard-Madoux, M.J.; Ober-Blöbaum, J.L.; Costes, L.M.; Kel, J.M.; Lindenbergh-Kortleve, D.J.; Brouwers-Haspels, I.; Heikema, A.P.; Samsom, J.N.; Clausen, B.E. IL-10 control of CD11c+ myeloid cells is essential to maintain immune homeostasis in the small and large intestine. *Oncotarget* **2016**, *7*, 32015–32030. [CrossRef]
33. Kühn, R.; Löhler, J.; Rennick, D.; Rajewsky, K.; Müller, W. Interleukin-10-deficient mice develop chronic enterocolitis. *Cell* **1993**, *75*, 263–274. [CrossRef]
34. Cardoso, A.; Gil Castro, A.; Martins, A.C.; Carriche, G.M.; Murigneux, V.; Castro, I.; Cumano, A.; Vieira, P.; Saraiva, M. The Dynamics of Interleukin-10-Afforded Protection during Dextran Sulfate Sodium-Induced Colitis. *Front. Immunol.* **2018**, *9*, 400. [CrossRef] [PubMed]
35. Steidler, L.; Hans, W.; Schotte, L.; Neirynck, S.; Obermeier, F.; Falk, W.; Fiers, W.; Remaut, E. Treatment of murine colitis by Lactococcus lactis secreting interleukin-10. *Science* **2000**, *289*, 1352–1355. [CrossRef] [PubMed]
36. Kim, S.C.; Tonkonogy, S.L.; Albright, C.A.; Tsang, J.; Balish, E.J.; Braun, J.; Huycke, M.M.; Sartor, R.B. Variable phenotypes of enterocolitis in interleukin 10-deficient mice monoassociated with two different commensal bacteria. *Gastroenterology* **2005**, *128*, 891–906. [CrossRef]
37. Schreiber, S.; Fedorak, R.N.; Nielsen, O.H.; Wild, G.; Williams, C.N.; Nikolaus, S.; Jacyna, M.; Lashner, B.A.; Gangl, A.; Rutgeerts, P.; et al. Safety and efficacy of recombinant human interleukin 10 in chronic active Crohn's disease. Crohn's Disease IL-10 Cooperative Study Group. *Gastroenterology* **2000**, *119*, 1461–1472.
38. Braat, H.; Rottiers, P.; Hommes, D.W.; Huyghebaert, N.; Remaut, E.; Remon, J.P.; van Deventer, S.J.; Neirynck, S.; Peppelenbosch, M.P.; Steidler, L. A phase I trial with transgenic bacteria expressing interleukin 10 in Crohn's disease. *Clin. Gastroenterol. Hepatol.* **2006**, *4*, 754–759. [CrossRef]
39. Olingampalli, K.L.; Balaji, S.; Wang, X.; Parikh, U.M.; Kaul, A.; Gilley, J.; Birla, R.K.; Bollyky, P.L.; Keswani, S.G. The Role of an IL-10/Hyaluronan Axis in Dermal Wound Healing. *Front. Cell Dev. Biol.* **2020**, *8*, 636. [CrossRef]
40. Leung, A.; Crombleholme, T.M.; Keswani, S.G. Fetal wound healing: Implications for minimal scar formation. *Curr. Opin. Pediatr.* **2012**, *24*, 371–378. [CrossRef] [PubMed]
41. Kieran, I.; Knock, A.; Bush, J.; So, K.; Metcalfe, A.; Hobson, R.; Mason, T.; O'Kane, S.; Ferguson, M. Interleukin-10 reduces scar formation in both animal and human cutaneous wounds: Results of two preclinical and phase II randomized control studies. *Wound Repair. Regen.* **2013**, *21*, 428–436. [CrossRef]
42. Yu, C.; Shan, T.; Feng, A.; Li, Y.; Zhu, W.; Xie, Y.; Li, N.; Li, J. Triptolide ameliorates Crohn's colitis is associated with inhibition of TLRs/NF-κB signaling pathway. *Fitoterapia* **2011**, *82*, 709–715. [CrossRef]
43. Deng, S.; Wang, A.; Chen, X.; Du, Q.; Wu, Y.; Chen, G.; Guo, W.; Li, Y. HBD Inhibits the Development of Colitis-Associated Cancer in Mice via the IL-6R/STAT3 Signaling Pathway. *Int. J. Mol. Sci.* **2019**, *20*, 1069. [CrossRef]

44. Yuan, K.; Li, X.; Lu, Q.; Zhu, Q.; Jiang, H.; Wang, T.; Huang, G.; Xu, A. Application and Mechanisms of Triptolide in the Treatment of Inflammatory Diseases—A Review. *Front. Pharmacol.* **2019**, *10*, 1469. [CrossRef] [PubMed]
45. Futagami, A.; Ishizaki, M.; Fukuda, Y.; Kawana, S.; Yamanaka, N. Wound healing involves induction of cyclooxygenase-2 expression in rat skin. *Lab. Investig.* **2002**, *82*, 1503–1513. [CrossRef]
46. Salgado, F.L.; Artigiani-Neto, R.; Lopes-Filho, G.D.J. Growth factors and cox2 in wound healing: An experimental study with ehrlich tumors. *Arq. Bras. Cir. Dig.* **2016**, *29*, 223–226. [CrossRef] [PubMed]
47. Yadav, V.P.; Shukla, A.; Choudhury, S.; Singh, R.; Anand, M.; Prabhu, S.N. IL1β/TNFα/COX-2/VEGF axis responsible for effective healing potential of C-glucoside xanthone (mangiferin) based ointment in immunocompromised rats. *Cytokine* **2002**, *158*, 156012. [CrossRef] [PubMed]
48. Hatazawa, R.; Tanaka, A.; Tanigami, M.; Amagase, K.; Kato, S.; Ashida, Y.; Takeuchi, K. Cyclooxygenase-2/prostaglandin E2 accelerates the healing of gastric ulcers via EP4 receptors. *Am. J. Physiol. Gastrointest. Liver Physiol.* **2007**, *293*, G788–G797. [CrossRef]
49. Wang, D.; DuBois, R.N. PPARδ and PGE2 signaling pathways communicate and connect inflammation to colorectal cancer. *Inflamm. Cell Signal* **2014**, *1*, 10.14800/ics.338. [CrossRef] [PubMed] [PubMed Central]
50. Riehl, T.E.; Alvarado, D.; Ee, X.; Ciorba, M.A.; Stenson, W.F. Hyaluronic acid promotes Lgr5+ stem cell proliferation and crypt fission through TLR4 and PGE2 transactivation of EGFR. *Am. J. Physiol. Gastrointest. Liver Physiol.* **2020**, *319*, G63–G73. [CrossRef] [PubMed]
51. Jackstadt, R.; Sansom, O.J. The Wae to repair: Prostaglandin E2 (PGE2) triggers intestinal wound repair. *EMBO J.* **2017**, *36*, 3–4. [CrossRef] [PubMed]
52. Miyoshi, H.; VanDussen, K.L.; Malvin, N.P.; Ryu, S.H.; Wang, Y.; Sonnek, N.M.; Lai, C.W.; Stappenbeck, T.S. Prostaglandin E2 promotes intestinal repair through an adaptive cellular response of the epithelium. *EMBO J.* **2017**, *36*, 5–24. [CrossRef]
53. Watanabe, T.; Kobata, A.; Tanigawa, T.; Nadatani, Y.; Yamagami, H.; Watanabe, K.; Tominaga, K.; Fujiwara, Y.; Takeuchi, K.; Arakawa, T. Activation of the MyD88 signaling pathway inhibits ischemia-reperfusion injury in the small intestine. *Am. J. Physiol. Gastrointest. Liver Physiol.* **2012**, *303*, G324–G334. [CrossRef]
54. Okayama, M.; Hayashi, S.; Aoi, Y.; Nishio, H.; Kato, S.; Takeuchi, K. Aggravation by selective COX-1 and COX-2 inhibitors of dextran sulfate sodium (DSS)-induced colon lesions in rats. *Dig. Dis. Sci.* **2007**, *52*, 2095–2103. [CrossRef]
55. Takeuchi, K.; Tanigami, M.; Amagase, K.; Ochi, A.; Okuda, S.; Hatazawa, R. Endogenous prostaglandin E2 accelerates healing of indomethacin-induced small intestinal lesions through upregulation of vascular endothelial growth factor expression by activation of EP4 receptors. *J. Gastroenterol. Hepatol.* **2010**, *25*, S67–S74. [CrossRef] [PubMed]
56. Baird, A.C.; Lloyd, F.; Lawrance, I.C. Prostaglandin E_2 and polyenylphosphatidylcholine protect against intestinal fibrosis and regulate myofibroblast function. *Dig. Dis. Sci.* **2015**, *60*, 1603–1616. [CrossRef] [PubMed]
57. Arron, M.N.; Lier, E.J.; de Wilt, J.H.; Stommel, M.W.; van Goor, H.; Ten Broek, R.P. Postoperative administration of non-steroidal anti-inflammatory drugs in colorectal cancer surgery does not increase anastomotic leak rate; A systematic review and meta-analysis. *Eur. J. Surg. Oncol.* **2020**, *46*, 2167–2217. [CrossRef] [PubMed]
58. Kastora, S.L.; Osborne, L.L.; Jardine, R.; Kounidas, G.; Carter, B.; Myint, P.K. Non-steroidal anti-inflammatory agents and anastomotic leak rates across colorectal cancer operations and anastomotic sites: A systematic review and meta-analysis of anastomosis specific leak rate and confounding factors. *Eur. J. Surg. Oncol.* **2021**, *47*, 2841–2848. [CrossRef] [PubMed]
59. Papafili, A.; Hill, M.R.; Brull, D.J.; McAnulty, R.J.; Marshall, R.P.; Humphries, S.E.; Laurent, G.J. Common promoter variant in cyclooxygenase-2 represses gene expression: Evidence of role in acute-phase inflammatory response. *Arterioscler. Thromb. Vasc. Biol.* **2002**, *22*, 1631–1636. [CrossRef]
60. Makar, K.W.; Poole, E.M.; Resler, A.J.; Seufert, B.; Curtin, K.; Kleinstein, S.E.; Duggan, D.; Kulmacz, R.J.; Hsu, L.; Whitton, J.; et al. COX-1 (PTGS1) and COX-2 (PTGS2) polymorphisms, NSAID interactions, and risk of colon and rectal cancers in two independent populations. *Cancer Causes Control* **2013**, *24*, 2059–2075. [CrossRef] [PubMed]
61. Perretti, M.; Getting, S.J.; Solito, E.; Murphy, P.M.; Gao, J.L. Involvement of the receptor for formylated peptides in the in vivo anti-migratory actions of annexin 1 and its mimetics. *Am. J. Pathol.* **2001**, *158*, 1969–1973. [CrossRef]
62. Belvedere, R.; Novizio, N.; Pessolano, E.; Tosco, A.; Eletto, D.; Porta, A.; Campiglia, P.; Perretti, M.; Filippelli, A.; Petrella, A. Heparan sulfate binds the extracellular Annexin A1 and blocks its effects on pancreatic cancer cells. *Biochem. Pharmacol.* **2020**, *182*, 114252. [CrossRef]
63. Sugimoto, M.A.; Vago, J.P.; Teixeira, M.M.; Sousa, L.P. Annexin A1 and the Resolution of Inflammation: Modulation of Neutrophil Recruitment, Apoptosis, and Clearance. *J. Immunol. Res.* **2016**, *2016*, 8239258. [CrossRef]
64. Babbin, B.A.; Parkos, C.A.; Mandell, K.J.; Winfree, L.M.; Laur, O.; Ivanov, A.I.; Nusrat, A. Annexin 2 regulates intestinal epithelial cell spreading and wound closure through Rho-related signaling. *Am. J. Pathol.* **2007**, *170*, 951–966. [CrossRef] [PubMed]
65. Fenteany, G.; Janmey, P.A.; Stossel, T. P Signaling pathways and cell mechanics involved in wound closure by epithelial cell sheets. *Curr. Biol.* **2000**, *10*, 831–838. [CrossRef]
66. Dalli, J.; Norling, L.V.; Renshaw, D.; Cooper, D.; Leung, K.Y.; Perretti, M. Annexin 1 mediates the rapid anti-inflammatory effects of neutrophil-derived microparticles. *Blood* **2008**, *112*, 2512–2519. [CrossRef] [PubMed]
67. Babbin, B.A.; Lee, W.Y.; Parkos, C.A.; Winfree, L.M.; Akyildiz, A.; Perretti, M.; Nusrat, A. Annexin I regulates SKCO 15 cell invasion by signaling through formyl peptide receptors. *J. Biol. Chem.* **2006**, *281*, 19588–19599. [CrossRef] [PubMed]

68. de Paula-Silva, M.; da Rocha, G.H.O.; Broering, M.F.; Queiroz, M.L.; Sandri, S.; Loiola, R.A.; Oliani, S.M.; Vieira, A.; Perretti, M.; Farsky, S.H.P. Formyl Peptide Receptors and Annexin A1: Complementary Mechanisms to Infliximab in Murine Experimental Colitis and Crohn's Disease. *Front. Immunol.* **2021**, *12*, 714138. [CrossRef]
69. de Paula-Silva, M.; Barrios, B.E.; Macció-Maretto, L.; Sena, A.A.; Farsky, S.H.P.; Correa, S.G.; Oliani, S.M. Role of the protein annexin A1 on the efficacy of anti-TNF treatment in a murine model of acute colitis. *Biochem. Pharmacol.* **2016**, *115*, 104–113. [CrossRef] [PubMed]
70. Hua, G.; He, C.; Lv, X.; Fan, L.; Wang, C.; Remmenga, S.W.; Rodabaugh, K.J.; Yang, L.; Lele, S.M.; Yang, P.; et al. The four and a half LIM domains 2 (FHL2) regulates ovarian granulosa cell tumor progression via controlling AKT1 transcription. *Cell Death Dis.* **2016**, *7*, e2297. [CrossRef]
71. Wixler, V. The role of FHL2 in wound healing and inflammation. *FASEB J.* **2019**, *33*, 7799–7809. [CrossRef] [PubMed]
72. Verset, L.; Feys, L.; Trépant, A.L.; De Wever, O.; Demetter, P. FHL2: A scaffold protein of carcinogenesis, tumour-stroma interactions and treatment response. *Histol. Histopathol.* **2016**, *31*, 469–478.
73. Friedrich, F.W.; Reischmann, S.; Schwalm, A.; Unger, A.; Ramanujam, D.; Münch, J.; Müller, O.J.; Hengstenberg, C.; Galve, E.; Charron, P.; et al. FHL2 expression and variants in hypertrophic cardiomyopathy. *Basic. Res. Cardiol.* **2014**, *109*, 451. [CrossRef]
74. Dao, D.T.; Anez-Bustillos, L.; Adam, R.M.; Puder, M.; Bielenberg, D.R. Heparin-Binding Epidermal Growth Factor-Like Growth Factor as a Critical Mediator of Tissue Repair and Regeneration. *Am. J. Pathol.* **2018**, *188*, 2446–2456. [CrossRef] [PubMed]
75. Pillai, S.B.; Hinman, C.E.; Luquette, M.H.; Nowicki, P.T.; Besner, G.E. Heparin-binding epidermal growth factor-like growth factor protects rat intestine from ischemia/reperfusion injury. *J. Surg. Res.* **1999**, *87*, 225–231. [CrossRef] [PubMed]
76. Yang, X.; Zhu, M.J.; Sreejayan, N.; Ren, J.; Du, M. Angiotensin II promotes smooth muscle cell proliferation and migration through release of heparin-binding epidermal growth factor and activation of EGF-receptor pathway. *Mol. Cells* **2005**, *20*, 263–270. [CrossRef] [PubMed]
77. Feng, J.; Besner, G.E. Heparin-binding epidermal growth factor-like growth factor promotes enterocyte migration and proliferation in neonatal rats with necrotizing enterocolitis. *J. Pediatr. Surg.* **2007**, *42*, 214–220. [CrossRef] [PubMed]
78. Xia, G.; Lara-Marquez, M.; Luquette, M.H.; Glenn, S.; Haque, A.; Besner, G.E. Heparin-binding EGF-like growth factor decreases inducible nitric oxide synthase and nitric oxide production after intestinal ischemia/reperfusion injury. *Antioxid. Redox Signal* **2001**, *3*, 919–930. [CrossRef]
79. El-Assal, O.N.; Radulescu, A.; Besner, G.E. Heparin-binding EGF-like growth factor preserves mesenteric microcirculatory blood flow and protects against intestinal injury in rats subjected to hemorrhagic shock and resuscitation. *Surgery* **2007**, *142*, 234–242. [CrossRef] [PubMed]
80. El-Assal, O.N.; Besner, G.E. HB-EGF enhances restitution after intestinal ischemia/reperfusion via PI3K/Akt and MEK/ERK1/2 activation. *Gastroenterology* **2005**, *129*, 609–625. [CrossRef]
81. Mehta, V.B.; Besner, G.E.; Mehta, V.B.; Besner, G.E. HB-EGF promotes angiogenesis in endothelial cells via PI3-kinase and MAPK signaling pathways. *Growth Factors* **2007**, *25*, 253–263. [CrossRef] [PubMed]
82. Dvorak, B.; Khailova, L.; Clark, J.A.; Hosseini, D.M.; Arganbright, K.M.; Reynolds, C.A.; Halpern, M.D. Comparison of epidermal growth factor and heparin-binding epidermal growth factor-like growth factor for prevention of experimental necrotizing enterocolitis. *J. Pediatr. Gastroenterol. Nutr.* **2008**, *47*, 11–18. [CrossRef]
83. Banerjee, A.; Schambach, F.; DeJong, C.S.; Hammond, S.M.; Reiner, S.L. Micro-RNA-155 inhibits IFN-gamma signaling in CD4+ T cells. *Eur. J. Immunol.* **2010**, *40*, 225–231. [CrossRef]

Journal of *Personalized Medicine*

MDPI

Systematic Review

HER2 Overexpression in Periampullary Tumors According to Anatomical and Histological Classification—A Systematic Review

Ioan Cătălin Bodea [1,2], Andra Ciocan [1,2,*], Florin Vasile Zaharie [1,2], Raluca Bodea [2], Florin Graur [1,2], Ștefan Ursu [1,2], Răzvan Alexandru Ciocan [3] and Nadim Al Hajjar [1,2]

1 Department of Surgery, "Iuliu Hațieganu" University of Medicine and Pharmacy, Croitorilor Street, No. 19–21, 400162 Cluj-Napoca, Romania; bodea_ioan_catalin@elearn.umfcluj.ro (I.C.B.); zaharie.vasile@umfcluj.ro (F.V.Z.); florin.graur@umfcluj.ro (F.G.); ursu_stefan@elearn.umfcluj.ro (Ș.U.); nadim.alhajjar@umfcluj.ro (N.A.H.)

2 "Octavian Fodor" Regional Institute of Gastroenterology and Hepatology, Croitorilor Street, No. 19–21, 400162 Cluj-Napoca, Romania; ralucabodea@yahoo.com

3 Department of Surgery-Practical Abilities, "Iuliu Hațieganu" University of Medicine and Pharmacy, Marinescu Street, No. 23, 400337 Cluj-Napoca, Romania; razvan.ciocan@umfcluj.ro

* Correspondence: andra.ciocan@umfcluj.ro

Abstract: Pancreatic cancer is one of the most aggressive, heterogeneous, and fatal types of human cancer; therefore, more effective therapeutic drugs are urgently needed. Human epidermal growth factor receptor 2 (HER2) overexpression and amplification have been identified as a cornerstone in this pathology. The aim of this review is to identify HER2 membrane overexpression in relation to pancreatic cancer pathways that can be used in order to develop a targeted therapy. After searching the keywords, 174 articles were found during a time span of 10 years, between 2013 and 2023, but only twelve scientific papers were qualified for this investigation. The new era of biomolecular research found a significant relationship between HER2 overexpression and pancreatic cancer cells in 25–30% of cases. The variables are dependent on tumor-derived cells, with differences in receptor overexpression between PDAC (pancreatic ductal adenocarcinoma), BTC (biliary tract cancer), ampullary carcinoma, and PNETs (pancreatic neuroendocrine tumors). HER2 overexpression is frequently encountered in human pancreatic carcinoma cell lines, and the ERBB family is one of the targets in the near future of therapy, with good results in phase I, II, and III studies evaluating downregulation and tumor downstaging, respectively.

Keywords: pancreatic cancer; protein receptors; HER2; overexpression; molecular pathway

1. Introduction

Pancreatic cancer (PC) is the seventh leading cause of cancer-related deaths worldwide, comprising 2.5% of all forms of cancer [1]. However, the heterogeneity of the disease makes the incidence higher in developed countries. The reasons for the vast differences in mortality rates of periampullary tumors are not yet completely understood, but they may be due to a lack of appropriate diagnosis, treatment, and follow-up [1]. Periampullary tumors are a widely used term to define a heterogeneous group of neoplasms deriving from completely different types of primordial cells: head of the pancreas (PDAC/PNET), distal common bile duct (BTC), and ampulla of Vater (ampullary carcinoma). This term should be correctly distinguished from ampullary carcinoma, or ampulloma, which is a tumor topographically centered in the region of the ampulla of Vater, deriving from the duodenal mucosal cells. Despite accounting for less than 10% of the total length of the small intestine, the duodenum, especially D2 (the second portion of it), is the site of 25% to 45% of all small bowel cancers. Ampullary carcinoma is a relatively uncommon neoplasm that accounts for approximately 6% of the total periampullary malignancies, with an incidence estimated at

2.9 cases per million in the general population and accounting for approximately 0.2% of gastrointestinal tract carcinomas. Distal cholangiocarcinoma is a rare malignancy of the biliary tract, occurring in 27% of total extrahepatic biliary adenocarcinomas [1,2]. With a 5-year survival rate of only 9% for pancreatic cancer and even lower depending on the histopathological type [2], this neoplasia caused 432, 242 new deaths in 2018 alone, and 458,918 new cases of pancreatic cancer are diagnosed every year [2,3]. To date, the etiology of pancreatic carcinoma is still insufficiently described due to the multitude of incriminating factors, although certain risk factors have been identified, such as diabetes mellitus, tobacco, dietary elements, alcohol abuse, obesity, age, ethnicity, family history, genetic factors, Helicobacter pylori infection, non-0 blood group, and chronic pancreatitis [4]. Surgery remains the main curative treatment, but only 15–20% of tumors are resectable at the time of diagnosis, and the prognosis is still poor, even for R0 resections [5–7]. Adjuvant chemotherapy seems to provide moderate improvements, with a medium survival of about 12 months; the regimen has not yet established favorable results [8,9]. Therefore, it is imperative to provide targeted therapy in order to improve overall and disease-free survival. Multiple studies are searching for the key components of protein receptors in the abnormal proliferation of neoplastic cells. Growth factors are essential for the development, growth, and homeostasis of multicellular organisms. Acting through cell surface receptors, growth factors are required for cell-to-cell communication, sustaining embryonic tissue induction, cell survival, apoptosis, tissue specialization, and cell migration. The epidermal growth factor family consists of four members: EGFR (ErbB1, HER1), ErbB2 (HER2, neu in rodents), ErbB3 (HER3), and ErbB4 (HER4). ErbB2, however, is unique in that it has no known ligand but is the preferred dimerization partner for other EGFRs [6,7]. *HER2* is a protooncogene located on chromosome 17 at q21 that encodes epidermal growth factor receptors with tyrosine kinase activity. In breast cancer, the *HER2* gene is amplified in 15%–20% of invasive breast cancers, and its amplification is closely linked to HER2 protein overexpression [10]. *HER2* amplification is a poor prognostic factor associated with a high rate of recurrence and mortality and is a predictive factor for response to certain chemotherapies [1,2]. Most importantly, it is a sole predictive marker for treatment benefits from HER2-targeting agents such as trastuzumab, lapatinib, and pertuzumab. As HER2-targeted therapy is exclusively effective in HER2-overexpressed and/or HER2-amplified breast cancers, precise assessment of HER2 status is an essential step in breast cancer treatment. The role of *HER2* in digestive tumors regarding both prognostic and therapeutic purposes provides heterogeneous results [11,12]. Novel testing and treatment guidelines are introducing HER2 evaluation in gastric and colorectal cancer, but for periampullary tumors, this protein receptor is less investigated. The rate of HER2 positivity in BTC (biliary tract cancers) has been reported to be 5–20% and between 5–50% for PDAC (pancreatic ductal adenocarcinoma). Case reports and clinical trials declare a good response to HER2 inhibitors as a treatment strategy, with abnormal cell proliferation reduction and tumor downstaging [10,13–15]. Above all carcinogenic pathways, the *HER2* pathway seems to be one of the most underestimated and undiagnosed protein receptors in pancreatic cancer. The main scope of this study is to bring together all the available information regarding HER2 overexpression in relation to tumor type, pancreatic ductal adenocarcinoma, distal cholangiocarcinoma, and ampullary tumor. Its overexpression and gene amplification are involved in tumor growth by cell proliferation and cell differentiation from normal into neoplastic ones [16–20]. HER2 lacks specific ligands, so it can form heterodimers only when activated by another receptor, such as EGFR, HER3, and HER4. In addition to abnormal overexpression, this receptor is able to spontaneously homodimerize, compared to HER3 or HER4 [21,22]. Worldwide, research attempts exist to identify the exact role of this receptor in abnormal cell proliferation in pancreatic cancer and periampullary tumors in general for anti-HER2 targeted therapy development. There is no standard therapy at the moment for HER2-positive pancreatic cancer patients, and this is the reason for our focus.

The aim of this review is to identify the overexpression of the HER2 protein receptor in relation to cephalopancreatic cancer and periampullary tumors in order to find out its role in cell proliferation. Consequently, the systematic review follows two trends of research—the role of the *HER2* pathway in pancreatic carcinogenesis and the rate of HER2 positivity according to the following tumor subtypes: pancreatic adenocarcinoma, distal cholangiocarcinoma, and ampullary carcinoma.

2. Materials and Methods

The methodology of this systematic review consists of defining search algorithms, selection criteria, and data extraction protocols. The present research followed the guidelines outlined in the Preferred Reporting Items for Systematic Reviews and Meta-Analyses (PRISMA) statement (Figure 1). From January 2013 until December 2023, articles published in English in the online databases PubMed (Medline), Embase, and Clarivate Web of Science were analyzed. This systematic review has not been registered.

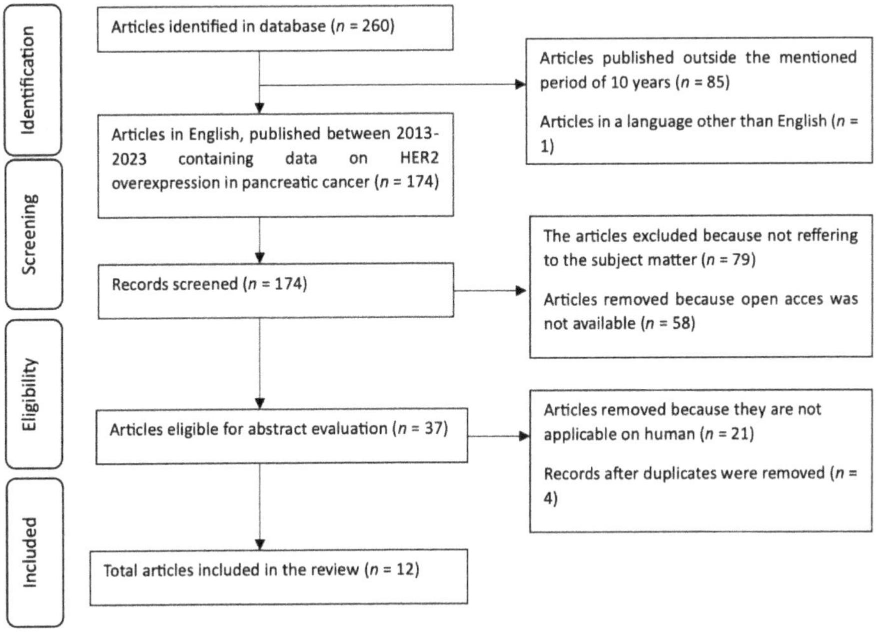

Figure 1. PRISMA flow diagram for the selected studies included in the systematic review identified in three databases, i.e., PubMed, Embase, and Clarivate Web of Science.

The research was performed using the following keywords: "pancreatic cancer" AND "protein receptors" AND "HER2" using "AND" and "OR" between the mentioned elements as Boolean operators. All titles referred to in English and published over a precise period of 10 years were assessed for eligibility by title and abstract by three separate researchers to reduce bias.

The inclusion criteria follow studies containing information about HER2 overexpression, the HER2 pathway, protein receptors in pancreatic cancer, distal cholangiocarcinoma, ampullary carcinoma, and pancreatic carcinogenesis. All studies were conducted on human cell lines. Exclusion criteria meant articles published earlier in 2013, not referring to the subject, letters to the editor, short reports, narrative reviews, non-English papers, articles focusing on *HER2* in other types of cancer (such as breast cancer, gastric cancer, and colorectal cancer), studies about other pathways in pancreatic cancer, and studies focusing on therapeutic effects on different cell lines and cell proliferation. For the risk of bias evaluation, we applied the updated quality assessment for diagnostic accuracy studies-2 (QUADAS-2) method to each article selected for analysis. It covered five areas of bias:

patient selection, index test, reference standard, subject flow, and timing. Microsoft Excel's extraction tool was used for data collection and database settlement. For the quality evaluation, we utilized standardized criteria, including study participation, factor measurement, value, and applicability. In the process of data selection and extraction, any inconsistencies identified by the three primary reviewers were subjected to further examination by two additional ones. The list of references for specific research projects was systematically examined to identify potential publications, following the snowball technique.

Using the above-mentioned keywords for search, 260 articles were found. By reducing the timeframe to 10 years, from 2013 until 2023, a number of 175 articles containing data on pancreatic cancer, cholangiocarcinoma, ampullary carcinoma, receptors, and HER2 were found. From this selection of articles, 1 article was removed because it was not written in English, and 79 were removed because they were not referring to the subject matter. Furthermore, 21 studies were excluded because they did not involve human subjects. A total of 58 articles were discarded because they were not open access. Moreover, 4 articles were removed because they were duplicates between the databases; therefore, 12 scientific papers remained eligible for the systematic review.

This systematic review has several limitations, mainly linked to inter-study heterogeneity. In some articles, a clear definition of the primary tumor site was not available, or the results were not reported separately for each subgroup, thus limiting the eligible data for inclusion in subgroup analysis. Since there are no standardized techniques and scores to assess HER2 amplification and expression available in PC and because there are no internationally established and validated methods for HER2 testing in any type of tumor, inconsistency in methodology may be an important issue. Differences in methodology, disease stage (early vs. advanced), tumor specimen (resection specimen vs. biopsy), site of tumor specimen (primary vs. metastatic), and IHC and ISH technical issues may explain the wide range of HER2 expression rate (1.1% to 76%) reported in this review. Finally, no survival data were available, making it impossible to assess the prognostic implications of HER2 overexpression or amplification.

3. Results

All articles included in the study (n = 12) focused on identifying the overexpression of the HER2 protein receptor in different cancer cell lines in relation to the histopathological type and possible upcoming targeted therapies. Among the evaluated articles, there were different HER2 determinations applied to inhomogeneous cohorts. All articles used human tissue or human cell lines obtained either by EUS (endoscopic ultrasound) biopsy—FNAC (fine needle aspiration cytology)—or resected samples after pancreatoduodenectomies. Protein receptor pathways involved in periampullary tumor development were analyzed, including the entire epidermal growth factor family, with a focus on HER2 overexpression and amplification, in order to provide quality data regarding targeted therapy against these dreadful tumors.

Each article examined a certain member of the growth family, like EGF, EGFR, HER1, HER2, HER3, and HER4, in accordance with a certain tumoral subtype; their aim is shown in Table 1.

Table 1. Author, year of publication, title of the article, and aim of the study.

Authors	Year of Publication	Title	Aim of the Study
Bittoni et al. [23]	2015	HER family Receptor Expression and Prognosis in Pancreatic Cancer	Identifying HER family overexpression in PDAC
Nicola et al. [24]	2016	HER2 aberrations and heterogeneity in cancers of the digestive system: Implications for pathologists and gastroenterologists	Identifying HER2 aberrations and overexpression in periampullary tumors

Table 1. *Cont.*

Authors	Year of Publication	Title	Aim of the Study
Xiaoping et al. [25]	2016	Prognostic role of HER2 amplification based on fluorescence in situ hybridization (FISH) in pancreatic ductal adenocarcinoma (PDAC): a meta-analysis	Identifying the prognostic role of HER2 positivity in PDAC
Elebro et al. [26]	2016	Expression and Prognostic Significance of Human Epidermal Growth Factor Receptors 1, 2 and 3 in Periampullary Adenocarcinoma	Identifying EGFR, HER2, and HER3 expression and HER2 amplification status in periampullary tumors
Salvatore et al. [27]	2017	HER2/HER3 pathway in biliary tract malignancies; systematic review and meta-analysis: a potential therapeutic target?	Identifying the HER2 overexpression rate in BTC
Majid et al. [28]	2019	The ERBB receptor inhibitor dacomitinib suppresses proliferation and invasion of pancreatic ductal adenocarcinoma cells	Evaluating dacomitinib's effect upon EGFR, HER2, and HER3 expression in PDAC
Assenat et al. [29]	2020	Phase II study evaluating the association of gemcitabine, trastuzumab and erlotinib as first-line treatment in patients with metastatic pancreatic adenocarcinoma (GATE 1)	Evaluating survival rate in patients with HER2+ advanced PDAC
Tanzeel et al. [30]	2020	Synergistic activity of agents targeting growth factor receptors, CDKs and downstream signaling molecules in a panel of pancreatic cancer cell lines and the identification of antagonistic combinations: Implications for future clinical trials in pancreatic cancer	Identifying cells' surface expression of various growth factor receptors in PDAC
Rabia et al. [31]	2021	Anti-tumoral activity of the Pan-HER (Sym013) antibody mixture in gemcitabine-resistant pancreatic cancer models	Identifying and understanding the pathways of the pan-HER antibody family in PDAC
Marinovic et al. [32]	2022	Analysis of polymorphisms in EGF, EGFR and *HER2* genes in pancreatic neuroendocrine tumors (PNETs)	Identifying the overexpression of EGF, EGFR, and HER2 receptors in PNET
Akihiro et al. [33]	2022	Multicenter phase II trial of trastuzumab deruxtecan for HER2-positive unresectable or recurrent biliary tract cancer: HERB trial	Identifying the benefit of trastuzumab deruxtecan on the ORR in HER2-positive BTC
de Vries et al. [34]	2023	Phase II study (KAMELEON) of single-agent T-DM1 in patients with HER2-positive advanced urothelial bladder cancer or pancreatic cancer/cholangiocarcinoma	Identifying the relationship between biomarkers and tumor response to treatment in PDAC and BTC

HER2, human epidermal growth factor receptor 2; HER3, human epidermal growth factor receptor 3; EGFR, epidermal growth factor receptor; ORR, objective response rate; T-DM1, antibody-drug conjugate trastuzumab emtansine; FISH, fluorescence in situ hybridization; PDAC, pancreatic ductal adenocarcinoma; BTC, biliary tract cancer; CDKs, cyclin-dependent kinase inhibitors; PNET, pancreatic neuroendocrine tumors.

Akihiro et al. [33] have demonstrated an overexpression rate of 10–20% for HER2 in biliary tree carcinomas, making trastuzumab–deruxtecan more active than FOLFIRINOX in difficult-to-treat, unresponsive, and HER2-expressing cases (Table 2). In addition, Majid et al. [28] demonstrated that dacomitinib, an irreversible tyrosine kinase inhibitor, exhibits stronger anti-tumor efficacy than single-targeted ERBB inhibitors in PDAC. Tanzel et al. [30] identified that afatinib in combination with the insulin-like growth factor 1 receptor (IGF-IR) inhibitor NVP-AEW541 resulted in a synergistic growth inhibition of pancreatic cancer cells. Assenat et al. [29] show that combining gemcitabine, trastuzumab, and erlotinib is more effective in terms of disease control rate, progression-free survival, and overall survival. The present systematic review reveals that sole inhibition of HER2 may not be enough because of the consequent upregulation of other ERBB family members, which can stimulate abnormal cell proliferation. In their study, Elebro et al. [26] demonstrated that the HER2-HER3 homodimer is a powerful activator of the PI3K/Akt pathway, causing aberrant proliferative and antiapoptotic intracellular signals. Inhibition of HER2 activity, however, causes upregulation of HER3, so simultaneous blockage of HER2 and HER3 activity gives more potent tumor cell inhibition than one receptor blockage alone.

Table 2. Authors, pathways targeted, drug agents used, number of patients related to carcinoma type, and detection methods used.

Authors	Pathways and Drugs Used	Number of Patients	Detection Method
Bittoni et al. [23]	N.A.	91 PDAC	IHC 1+
Nicola et al. [24]	Topoisomerase inhibition Trastuzumab deruxtecan + Capecitabine	17 PDAC	IHC2+ and 3+ ISH 2+ and 3+
Xiaoping et al. [25]	N.A.	764 PDAC	ISH 1+ and 2+
Elebro et al. [26]	N.A.	175 PDAC + BTC + AVC	(TMAs) IHC 2+ and 3+
Salvatore et al. [27]	N.A.	920 BTC 303 AVC	IHC2+ and 3+ ISH 2+ and 3+
Majid et al. [28]	ERBB inhibition Dacomitinib + lapatinib	96 PDAC	MTT assay
Assenat et al. [29]	Tyrosine kinase inhibition Erlotinib + Trastuzumab + Gemcitabine	62 PDAC	IHC 2+ and 3+
Tanzeel et al. [30]	Tyrosine kinase inhibition Dinaciclib + afatinib + dasatinib	96 PDAC	Flow cytometry (fluorescence intensity MFI)
Rabia et al. [31]	Pan-HER Inhibition	45 PDAC (Gemcitabine-resistant cells)	IHC 2+ and 3+
Marinovic et al. [32]	N.A.	68 PNETs	SNP genotyping
Akihiro et al. [33]	Topoisomerase inhibition Trastuzumab deruxtecan	32 BTC	IHC 2+ and 3+ ISH 2+ and 3+
de Vries et al. [34]	Topoisomerase inhibition Trastuzumab emtansine	133 PDAC 82 BTC	IHC 3+

SNP, single nucleotide polymorphism; TMAs, tissue microarrays; MTT assay, cell metabolic activity; FISH, fluorescence in situ hybridization; IHC, immunohistochemistry; PNETs, pancreatic neuroendocrine tumors; PDAC, pancreatic ductal adenocarcinoma; BTC, biliary tract cancer/cholangiocarcinoma; AVC, ampulla of Vater carcinoma.

Regarding the pathways targeted and drug agents used in their studies, authors favored topoisomerase inhibitors, panERBB receptor inhibitors and tyrosine kinase inhibitors to reduce cancer cell proliferation and increase survival (Table 3). The most frequently used inhibitory agent was trastuzumab. Tanzeel et al. [30] mentioned that the combination of dinaciclib, afatinib, and an insulin-like growth factor 1 receptor inhibitor is the most effective downstaging treatment in pancreatic cancer. Majid et al. [28] show that dacomitinib induces cell apoptosis in PDAC by inhibiting XIAP, cIAP1, and cIAP2.

Table 3. Author and significant therapeutic findings.

Title	Immunotherapy vs. Chemotherapy in *HER2+*
Bittoni et al. [23]	Trastuzumab + Capecitabine > Capecitabine alone in PDAC

Table 3. *Cont.*

Title	Immunotherapy vs. Chemotherapy in *HER2*+
Nicola et al. [24]	Trastuzumab-emtansine + Gemcitabine > Gemcitabine alone in BTC and metastatic digestive tumors
Xiaoping et al. [25]	Trastuzumab + gemcitabine > chemotherapy + gemcitabine in PDAC
Elebro et al. [26]	Erlotinib + gemcitabine > chemotherapy + gemcitabine in BTC and PDAC
Salvatore et al. [27]	Pertuzumab + trastuzumab/pertuzumab emtansine + Gemcitabine > Cisplatin + gemcitabine in BTC
Majid et al. [28]	Afatinib > erlotinib in PDAC
Assenat et al. [29]	FOLFIRINOX > Trastuzumab + erlotinib + Gemcitabine > Nab-paclitaxel + gemcitabine in PDAC
Tanzeel et al. [30]	Afatinib + IGF-IR/afatinib + dasatinib/dasatinib + gemcitabine > chemotherapy + gemcitabine in PDAC
Rabia et al. [31]	Cetuximab + trastuzumab + pertuzumab > chemotherapy + gemcitabine in PDAC
Marinovic et al. [32]	Cetuximab + trastuzumab > Erlotinib + trastuzumab in PNET
Akihiro et al. [33]	Trastuzumab deruxtecan > FOLFOX/FOLFIRI in BTC
de Vries et al. [34]	Trastuzumab deruxtecan/trastuzumab duocarmazine + chemotherapy > chemotherapy alone in BTC

BTC, biliary tract cancer; PDAC, pancreatic ductal adenocarcinoma; PNET, pancreatic neuroendocrine tumors; >, better treatment outcome in terms of efficacy.

A large variation in the number of patients included in the cohorts evaluated in each study exists. Furthermore, there is no specific histopathological division between distal cholangiocarcinoma and suprapancreatic cholangiocarcinoma regarding BTC.

In pancreatic cancer, Rabia et al. [31] showed that simultaneous targeting of EGFR and *HER2* with cetuximab and trastuzumab induces a synergistic therapeutic effect. They extended their strategy by adding pertuzumab (an anti-HER2 antibody) to 9F7-F11 (an anti-HER3 antibody) in PDAC. The monoclonal antibody combination blocked MAPK and AKT pathways by disrupting hetero- and homodimers and induced receptor down-regulation.

Regarding the technique used for HER2 detection, 8 out of 12 authors used immunohistochemistry, i.e., Tanzeel et al. [30] used flow cytometry; Marinovic et al. [32] used SPN genotyping; Majid et al. [28] used MTT assay-cell metabolic activity; and Elebro et al. [26] used tissue microarrays (TMAs). Moreover, Akihiro, Nicola, and Salvatore used both IHC and ISH to reveal HER2 overexpression. The researchers struggle to find the best technique in terms of both qualitative and quantitative values, according to purpose and funds [24,27,33].

HER2 positivity rates vary largely from study to study, mainly due to the differences in sample quality and cohort size. Akihiro et al. [33] included 32 patients in their study, compared to Salvatore et al. [27], who conducted the research on 920 patients (Table 2). Consequently, HER2 positivity rates oscillate between 1.1 and 76% in PDAC, with an average of 30%, and 5 to 76% in BTC. For pancreatic neuroendocrine tumors, HER+ ranges between 35 and 40%, more than the median of PDAC. Marinovic et al. [32] found a median of 37.9% in nonfunctional neuroendocrine tumors and 36.11% in functional tumors (Table 4). Xiaoping et al. [25] discovered that in some samples there is not just one ERBB receptor of the family upregulated or overexpressed but two or three receptors, which co-stimulate abnormal cell proliferation. The authors determined HER2+ in 24% of PDAC cases and the combination of EGFR, HER2 2+, and HER3 2+ in 11%.

Table 4. Author, HER2+ expression and histopathological type, and drug agent.

Author	HER2 Overexpression According to Histopathological Type	Target Agents
Bittoni et al. [23]	1.1% in PDAC	Trastuzumab
Nicola et al. [24]	5–76% overexpression and 1–8% amplification in BTC 0–50% overexpression and 2–29% amplification in PDAC	Trastuzumab, Pertuzumab, Lapatinib, Neratinib, Afatinib

Table 4. *Cont.*

Author	HER2 Overexpression According to Histopathological Type	Target Agents
Xiaoping et al. [25]	2.1–23.8% overexpression and 16% amplification in PDAC	Trastuzumab
Elebro et al. [26]	11% in PDAC 7% in BTC 15% in AVC	Erlotinib
Salvatore et al. [27]	19.9% in PDAC 17.4% in BTC 27.9% in AVC	Trastuzumab, Pertuzumab
Majid et al. [28]	16% in resectable PDAC 26% in metastatic PDAC	Dacomitinib
Assenat et al. [29]	58.3% in PDAC	Trastuzumab, Erlotinib
Tanzeel et al. [30]	26.27% in PDAC	Dinaciclib, Afatinib, IGF-IR
Rabia et al. [31]	24% in PDAC with 11% positive for combination of EGFR + *HER2* + HER3	Trastuzumab, Lapatinib, U3-1287
Marinovic et al. [32]	37.9% in nonfunctional PNET 36.11% in functional PNET 42.31% in insulinomas	Trastuzumab, Cetuximab
Akihiro et al. [33]	10–20% in BTC	Trastuzumab Deruxtecan
de Vries et al. [34]	6.3% in PDAC 7.9% in BTC	Trastuzumab Duocarmazine

BTC, biliary tract cancer; PDAC, pancreatic ductal adenocarcinoma; AVC, ampula of Vater cancer; U3-1287, anti-HER3 antibody; PNET, pancreatic neuroendocrine tumors; IGF-IR, insulin-like growth factor 1 receptor inhibitor.

Akihiro et al. showed that trastuzumab deruxtecan is more effective than standard chemotherapy (FOLFOX) in difficult-to-treat HER2+ cases of cholangiocarcinoma. In particular, trastuzumab has greatly improved the therapeutic approach of advanced BTC but has little evidence in other digestive cancers, as proved by Nicola et al. Trastuzumab in combination with cytotoxic therapies in HER2-positive BTC has increased the tumor response rate from 35% to 47%, improving progression-free survival from 5.5 months to 6.7 months and overall survival from 11.1 months to 13.8 months. The combination of pertuzumab and trastuzumab has been reported to induce a synergistic inhibition of in vivo tumor growth in BTC due to a more complex blockade of HER2/HER3 signaling, as shown in Salvatore et al. All chemo- and immunotherapics are thoroughly explained in File S1 from the Supplementary Materials.

Comparing trastuzumab plus chemotherapy versus chemotherapy alone, de Vries et al. showed an overall survival benefit with this combination instead of chemotherapy alone, regardless of variability in HER2 staining, with a numerically greater benefit in patients with less variable HER2 protein expression (>30% of stained cells), out of which only one patient with PDAC and two with BTC had strong HER2+ and 3+ tumors.

Assenat et al. proved that increased co-expression of EGFR and HER2 is associated with advanced tumor stage, aggressive phenotype, the presence of distant metastases, and shorter overall survival. Therefore, the combination of gemcitabine, trastuzumab, and erlotinib is more effective in terms of disease control rate, progression-free survival, and overall survival. The triplet has not reported unexpected toxicity results, except for a higher rate of thromboembolic complications (33%) than usually described in metastatic PDAC (15–20%), which is similar to the combination of gemcitabine and nab-paclitaxel.

In their study, Rabia et al. described that tumor resistance to gemcitabine is accompanied by HER2 and HER3 overexpression. Simultaneous targeting of EGFR and HER2 with cetuximab and trastuzumab induces a synergistic therapeutic effect. Afatinib is more effective than erlotinib in inhibiting growth factors in PDAC, more so in combination with the insulin-like growth factor 1 receptor (IGF-IR).

4. Discussion

Despite major advances in the early diagnosis of solid tumors in the past three decades, pancreatic cancer and distal cholangiocarcinoma, likewise, remain challenging in terms of curative treatment [35]. By 2030, it is predicted to become the second-leading cause of cancer-related deaths after lung cancer [36]. Due to their heterogeneous nature, retroperitoneal location, non-specific symptoms, and lack of screening methods, the overwhelming majority of cephalopancreatic tumors are diagnosed in advanced stages [37]. Until now, only a few HER inhibitors and EGFR-specific tyrosine kinase inhibitors (TKI), like erlotinib, lapatinib, and gefitinib, have gained FDA approval for the targeted therapy of locally advanced, unresectable, or metastatic pancreatic cancer in combination with the cytotoxic agent gemcitabine. Erlotinib and gefitinib are most effective on EGFR, and lapatinib is equally active against EGFR and HER2. Because of the late diagnosis and untargeted treatment, most of these patients have a low survival rate of 10% at 5 years from diagnosis. Almost 60–70% of PDAC cases are localized cephalopancreatic. It is mandatory to develop a good algorithm for neoadjuvant treatment for tumor downstaging and downsizing targeted at overexpressed receptor inhibition or downregulation. Similar to HER2+ therapy used in breast and gastric cancer with good results, the biomolecular substrate of pancreatic cancer may include HER2 targeted treatment. Since not only a single receptor is overexpressed in pancreatic cancer, additional information regarding ERBB is needed. This resides in the entire HER family expression analysis to be able to block the whole HER signaling network and increase the anti-tumor response. Most of the drug combinations effectively decrease cell proliferation in experimental animal models, but their clinical efficiency needs to be demonstrated [38–40].

The tyrosine kinase function of ERBB members is the key to intracellular signaling, activation, and cell transformation, which can work as target agents for tyrosine kinase inhibitors (TKIs). The binding characteristics of each TKI vary according to a specific EGFR mutation, and the choice of TKI agents is based on the unique molecular features of the tumor. Lapatinib connects to the inactive conformation of EGFR with a particularly tight binding that affords a slow off-rate [41]. In a study conducted by Akihiro et al., trastuzumab deruxtecan is the next TKI to be the standard second line of targeted treatment, proving benefit in HER2-positive unresectable or recurrent BTC. In a phase I study, trastuzumab deruxtecan led to an almost 80% reduction in tumor size in patients with distal cholangiocarcinoma. These data suggest that there may be promise in targeting HER2 in non-breast/non gastric carcinomas [28,42,43]. Chemo- and immunotherapy combinations provide better results in terms of EGFR-HER2 or HER2-HER3 heterodimer disorganization, more efficient and stable inhibition of signaling pathways, and increased degradation of HER2 receptors [16]. Afatinib, a pan-HER blocker, is more effective than erlotinib in inhibiting pancreatic cancer cell proliferation, as reported by Tanzeel et al. Furthermore, of all agents examined in their study, CDK1/2/5/9 inhibitor–dinaciclib was the most potent and effective agent against both primary and metastatic cell proliferation in all periampullary tumors. Improved survival of normal pancreatic cells, a high apoptosis rate, and enhanced radiosensitivity are shown by Majid et al. by treating the PDAC cells with dacomitinib. Moreover, it demonstrated that the anti-tumor activity of single-targeted ERBBs like cetuximab, trastuzumab, and erlotinib was marginal in downgrading the PDAC microenvironment. These hypotheses suggest that for better results, pan-ERBB inhibitors may yield stronger anti-tumoral activity than a single targeted ERBB agent.

Increased co-expression of EGFR and HER2 is associated with advanced tumor stages, aggressive phenotypes, distant metastases, and shorter overall survival. Furthermore, co-expression of HER3 and HER4 is associated with increased tumor size, advanced tumor stage, and high invasiveness [44,45]. Local tumor progression and early systemic dissemination of PDAC cells contribute to a bad prognosis, which is one of the major hallmarks of the disease. Elebro et al. reported that HER3 expression is a favorable prognostic factor in the ampulla of Vater carcinoma–intestinal type, and EGFR overexpression is an adverse one. In pancreato-biliary type, EGFR was found to be a negative prognostic factor, implying resistance to adjuvant gemcitabine [46]. Moreover, HER2 overexpression is an important prognostic factor both for the intestinal and pancreato-biliary types of periampullary tumors. Taking all this into consideration, their statistical significance is moderate when we consider these associations independent of other prognostic factors.

For pancreatic neuroendocrine tumors (PNETs), Marinovic et al. emphasized that the combination of EGF, EGFR, and HER2 plays a significant role in carcinogenesis and impacts susceptibility to various treatment strategies. EGFR overexpression is associated with aggressive types of gastrinoma-functional PNET, similar to PDAC. However, none of the variant genotypes of EGF, EGFR, or HER2 is associated with distant metastases. When it comes to HER2 overexpression in PNETs, there is equal dissemination between functional and nonfunctional tumors. Furthermore, insulinomas demonstrate approximately 42.31% HER2 positivity, higher than the median range, and they may be considered herapeutic targets in PNET because of their high incidence. Tanzeel et al. reported that CDK inhibitor dinaciclib, an irreversible pan-HER tyrosine kinase inhibitor afatinib, and SRC tyrosine kinase inhibitor dasatinib were the most effective agents, inhibiting cell proliferation and migration.

Because there are a multitude of pathological pathways and protein receptors, blocking just one pathway is not effective because carcinogenesis consists of a cumulation of biomolecular alterations; therefore, the use of agents in combination is the key.

For BTC, there is no specific difference between distal cholangiocarcinoma and main biliary duct tumors of the suprapancreatic area. There is no variation in protein receptors between the ampulla of Vater carcinomas and duodenal tumors invading the head of the pancreas. Salvatore et al. described a 17.4% positivity rate of HER2 overexpression in BTC and 27.9% in ampulla Vater carcinoma, in line with the median range of HER2+ in PDAC.

Regarding the method used for HER2 overexpression assay and analysis, IHC (immunohistochemistry) and ISH (in situ hybridization) are frequently used for formalin-fixed paraffin-embedded tissue. IHC measures the total number of HER2 receptors on the cell's surface for receptor overexpression quantification, and ISH detects the number of copies of the *HER2* gene evidenced in tumor cells' nuclei. Currently, there is no standard guideline for HER2 status evaluation in pancreatic cancer, hence the necessity to develop a standard procedure in order to efficiently compare results. Because of the heterogeneity of the cohorts and the lack of a standard HER2 assay method, it is hard to compare the results of multiple studies because they use different diagnostic methods.

Nagarkar et al. studied and presented a case report of HER2-positive distal common bile duct carcinoma with multiple relapses and overexpression of the *HER2* gene, which was used as a potential target to treat the patient with trastuzumab. The combination of trastuzumab with cyclophosphamide and methotrexate yielded an excellent treatment response, with the patient remaining in complete response until the last follow-up [47].

Before considering chemotherapy, a complete proteomic profile of overexpressed surface receptors in the cell membrane is necessary. For that, a preoperative biopsy is performed to analyze HER2 overexpression. Studying the effects of combining pan-HER with standard-of-care agents, such as gemcitabine or FOLFIRINOX, is essential. Specific targeted therapy is also needed to downregulate and decrease tumor burden in order to restore it to surgical resectability.

The limitation of the study resides in the fact that various articles provide heterogeneous results. They all convey that HER2 overexpression plays an important role in tumor growth, cell invasion, and proliferation, but with different statistical data. Elebro et al. show 58.3% of HER2+ in 62 patients, compared to a minimum rate of 2.1% found by Xiaoping et al. These major discrepancies come from the distinct cohorts in various articles, the lack of standard diagnostic protocols, and the HER2 overexpression analysis method, making the results difficult to compare between studies. Moreover, the sample size and quality might generate inconsistencies in IHC or ISH positivity.

5. Conclusions

Pancreatic cancer remains one of the deadliest cancer types worldwide. During carcinogenesis, HER2 has been identified as an oncogene involved in the upregulation of tumor cell proliferation and invasion. HER2 overexpression has been found in 20–30% of all periampullary tumors, highly dependent upon the histopathological type. Inhibiting the pan-ERBB receptors increases disease control and reduces PDAC growth, with a favorable prognosis. Combined chemotherapy and immunotherapy in HER2+ tumors is a new approach involving simultaneous targeting of each receptor pathway of the HER family. Therefore, HER2 overexpression should be routinely evaluated in cephalopancreatic adenocarcinomas, distal cholangiocarcinomas, and ampullary carcinomas prior to surgery or chemotherapy in order to have a correct indication for systemic treatment and provide targeted treatment.

Supplementary Materials: The following supporting information can be downloaded at: https://www.mdpi.com/article/10.3390/jpm14050463/s1, File S1: All Chemo- and Immunotherapics.

Author Contributions: Conceptualization, I.C.B., A.C. and N.A.H.; methodology, I.C.B., A.C., R.A.C. and F.G.; software, R.B. and F.G.; validation, N.A.H.; formal analysis, Ș.U. and R.A.C.; investigation, I.C.B., A.C. and Ș.U.; resources, R.B., F.V.Z., F.G. and N.A.H.; data curation, I.C.B., R.A.C. and Ș.U.; writing—original draft preparation, I.C.B. and Ș.U.; writing—review and editing, A.C., R.A.C. and N.A.H.; visualization, R.B., F.V.Z., F.G. and N.A.H.; supervision, N.A.H.; project administration, I.C.B., A.C. and N.A.H.; All authors have read and agreed to the published version of the manuscript.

Funding: 1. This research was funded by the "Iuliu Hațieganu" University of Medicine and Pharmacy Cluj-Napoca, Romania, Doctoral Research Program, through the project PCD 771/8/11.01.2023. 2. This work was granted by project PDI-PFE-CDI 2021, entitled Increasing the Performance of Scientific Research, Supporting Excellence in Medical Research and Innovation, PROGRES, No. 40PFE/30.12.2021.

Institutional Review Board Statement: Not applicable.

Informed Consent Statement: Not applicable.

Data Availability Statement: Data are contained within the article.

Acknowledgments: This research was supported by the project "New smart and adaptive robotics solutions for personalized minimally invasive surgery in cancer treatment—ATHENA", which was funded by the European Union—NextGenerationEU and the Romanian Government under the National Recovery and Resilience Plan for Romania, contract No. 760072/23.05.2023, code CF 16/15.11.2022.

Conflicts of Interest: The authors declare no conflicts of interest.

References

1. Hidalgo, M. Pancreatic cancer. *N. Engl. J. Med.* **2010**, *362*, 1605–1617. [PubMed]
2. Siegel, R.; Naishadham, D.; Jemal, A. Cancer statistics. *CA Cancer J. Clin.* **2012**, *62*, 10–29. [CrossRef] [PubMed]
3. Lowenfels, A.B.; Maisonneuve, P. Epidemiology and risk factors for pancreatic cancer. *Best Pract. Res. Clin. Gastroenterol.* **2006**, *20*, 197–209. [CrossRef]
4. Koorstra, J.B.; Hustinx, S.R.; Offerhaus, G.J.; Maitra, A. Pancreatic carcinogenesis. *Pancreatology* **2008**, *8*, 110–125. [CrossRef] [PubMed]
5. Beuran, M.; Negoi, I.; Paun, S.; Ion, A.D.; Bleotu, C.; Negoi, R.I.; Hostiuc, S. The epithelial to mesenchymal transition in pancreatic cancer: A systematic review. *Pancreatology* **2015**, *15*, 217–225. [CrossRef] [PubMed]
6. Hezel, A.F.; Kimmelman, A.C.; Stanger, B.Z.; Bardeesy, N.; Depinho, R.A. Genetics and biology of pancreatic ductal adenocarcinoma. *Genes Dev.* **2006**, *20*, 1218–1249. [CrossRef] [PubMed]
7. Garcea, G.; Neal, C.P.; Pattenden, C.J.; Steward, W.P.; Berry, D.P. Molecular prognostic markers in pancreatic cancer: A systematic review. *Eur. J. Cancer* **2005**, *41*, 2213–2236. [CrossRef] [PubMed]

8. Neoptolemos, J.P.; Stocken, D.D.; Bassi, C.; Ghaneh, P.; Cunningham, D.; Goldstein, D.; Padbury, R.; Moore, M.J.; Gallinger, S.; Mariette, C.; et al. Adjuvant chemotherapy with fluorouracil plus folinic acid vs. gemcitabine following pancreatic cancer resection: A randomized controlled trial. *JAMA* **2010**, *304*, 1073–1081. [CrossRef] [PubMed]
9. Ramanathan, R.K.; Belani, C.P.; Singh, D.A.; Tanaka, M.; Lenz, H.J.; Yen, Y.; Kindler, H.L.; Iqbal, S.; Longmate, J.; Mack, P.C.; et al. A phase II study of lapatinib in patients with advanced biliary tree and hepatocellular cancer. *Cancer Chemother. Pharmacol.* **2009**, *64*, 777–783. [CrossRef]
10. Moasser, M.M. The oncogene *HER2*: Its signaling and transforming functions and its role in human cancer pathogenesis. *Oncogene* **2007**, *26*, 6469–6487. [CrossRef]
11. Adsay, N.V.; Merati, K.; Basturk, O.; Iacpbuzio-Donahue, C.; Levi, E.; Cheng, J.D.; Sarkar, F.H.; Hruban, R.H.; Klimsta, D.S. Pathologically and biologically distinct types of epithelium in intraductal papillary mucinous neoplasms: Delineation of an "intestinal" pathway of carcinogenesis in the pancreas. *Am. J. Surg. Pathol.* **2004**, *28*, 839–848. [CrossRef]
12. Pignochino, Y.; Sarotto, I.; Peraldo-Neia, C.; Penachioni, J.Y.; Cavalloni, G.; Migliardi, G.; Casorzo, L.; Chiorino, G.; Risio, M.; Bardelli, A.; et al. Targeting EGFR/*HER2* pathways enhances the antiproliferative effect of gemcitabine in biliary tract and gallbladder carcinomas. *BMC Cancer.* **2010**, *10*, 631. [CrossRef]
13. Gerdes, B.; Wild, A.; Wittenberg, J.; Barth, P.; Ramaswamy, A.; Kersting, M.; Luttges, J.; Klöppel, G.; Bartsch, D.K. Tumor-suppressing pathways in cystic pancreatic tumors. *Pancreas* **2003**, *13*, 42–48. [CrossRef]
14. Roskoski, R. The ErbB/HER family of protein-tyrosine kinases and cancer. *Pharmacol. Res.* **2014**, *79*, 34–74. [CrossRef] [PubMed]
15. Aumayr, K.; Soleiman, A.; Sahora, K.; Schindl, M.; Werba, G.; Schoppmann, S.F.; Birner, P. *HER2* gene amplification and protein expression in pancreatic ductal adenocarcinomas. *Appl. Immunohistochem. Mol. Morphol.* **2014**, *22*, 146–152. [CrossRef]
16. Larbouret, C.; Robert, B.; Navarro-Teulon, I.; Thèzenas, S.; Ladjemi, M.-Z.; Morisseau, S.; Campigna, E.; Bibeau, F.; Mach, J.P.; Pèlegrin, A.; et al. In vivo Therapeutic synergism of anti-epidermal growth factor receptor and anti-*HER2* monoclonal antibodies against pancreatic carcinomas. *Clin. Cancer Res.* **2007**, *13*, 3356–3362. [CrossRef] [PubMed]
17. Ben-Kasus, T.; Schechter, B.; Lavi, S.; Yarden, Y.; Sela, M. Persistent elimination of ErbB-2/*HER2*-overexpressing tumors using combinations of monoclonal antibodies: Relevance of receptor endocytosis. *Proc. Natl. Acad. Sci. USA* **2009**, *106*, 3294–3299. [CrossRef] [PubMed]
18. Hynes, N.E.; Lane, H.A. ERBB receptors and cancer: The complexity of targeted inhibitors. *Nat. Rev. Cancer* **2005**, *5*, 341–354. [CrossRef]
19. Marks, E.I.; Yee, N.S. Molecular genetics and targeted therapeutics in biliary tract carcinoma. *World J. Gastroenterol.* **2016**, *22*, 1335–1347. [CrossRef]
20. Mendelsohn, J.; Baselga, J. The EGF receptor family as targets for cancer therapy. *Oncogene* **2000**, *19*, 6550–6565. [CrossRef]
21. Chow, N.H.; Huang, S.M.; Chan, S.H.; Mo, L.R.; Hwang, M.H.; Su, W.C. Significance of c-erbB-2 expression in normal and neoplastic epithelium of biliary tract. *Anticancer. Res.* **1995**, *15*, 1055–1059. [PubMed]
22. Collier, J.D.; Guo, K.; Mathew, J.; May, F.E.; Bennett, M.K.; Corbett, I.P.; Bassendine, M.F.; Burt, A.D. c-erbB-2 oncogene expression in hepatocellular carcinoma and cholangiocarcinoma. *J. Hepatol.* **1992**, *14*, 377–380. [CrossRef] [PubMed]
23. Bittoni, A.; Mandolesi, A.; Andrikou, K.; Santoni, M.; Alfonsi, S.; Lanese, A.; Loretelli, C.; Pellei, C.; Piva, F.; Scarpelli, M.; et al. HER family Receptor Expression and Prognosis in Pancreatic Cancer. *Int. J. Biol. Markers* **2015**, *30*, 327–332. [CrossRef] [PubMed]
24. Nicola, F.; Silvano, B. *HER2* aberrations and heterogeneity in cancers of the digestive system: Implications for pathologists and gastroenterologists. *World J. Gastroenterol.* **2016**, *22*, 7926–7937. [CrossRef] [PubMed]
25. Li, X.; Zhao, H.; Gu, J.; Zheng, L. Prognostic role of *HER2* amplification based on fluorescence in situ hybridization (FISH) in pancreatic ductal adenocarcinoma (PDAC): A meta-analysis. *World J. Surg. Oncol.* **2016**, *14*, 38. [CrossRef] [PubMed]
26. Elebro, J.; Heby, M.; Warfvinge, C.F.; Nodin, B.; Eberhard, J.; Jirstrom, K. Expression and Prognostic Significance of Human Epidermal Growth Factor Receptors 1, 2 and 3 in Periampullary Adenocarcinoma. *PLoS ONE* **2016**, *11*, 0153533. [CrossRef] [PubMed]
27. Galdy, S.; Lamarca, A.; McNamara, M.G.; Hubner, R.A.; Cella, C.A.; Fazio, N.; Valle, J.W. *HER2*/HER3 pathway in biliary tract malignancies; systematic review and meta-analysis: A potential therapeutic target? *Cancer Metastasis Rev.* **2017**, *36*, 141–157. [CrossRef] [PubMed]
28. Majid, M.; Fatemeh, E.; Sepideh, H.; Hassan, Y.; Sepehr, J.; Vasimeh, V.; Alishahi, Z.; Mousavipak, S.H.; Bashash, D.; Dehpour, A.R.; et al. The ERBB receptor inhibitor dacomitinib suppresses proliferation and invasion of pancreatic ductal adenocarcinoma cells. *Cell Oncol.* **2019**, *42*, 491–504. [CrossRef]
29. Assenat, E.; Mineur, L.; Mollevi, C.; Lopez-Crapez, E.; Lombard-Bohas, C.; Samalin, E.; Portales, F.; Walter, T.; de Forges, H.; Dupuy, M.; et al. Phase II study evaluating the association of gemcitabine, trastuzumab and erlotinib as first-line treatment in patients with metastatic pancreatic adenocarcinoma (GATE 1). *Int. J. Cancer* **2020**, *1*, 682–691. [CrossRef] [PubMed]
30. Khan, T.; Seddon, A.M.; Dalgleish, A.G.; Khelwatty, S.; Ioannou, N.; Mudan, S.; Modjtahedi, H. Synergistic activity of agents targeting growth factor receptors, CDKs and downstream signaling molecules in a panel of pancreatic cancer cell lines and the identification of antagonistic combinations: Implications for future clinical trials in pancreatic cancer. *Oncol. Rep.* **2020**, *44*, 2581–2594. [CrossRef]
31. Rabia, E.; Garambois, V.; Hubert, J.; Bruciamacchie, M.; Pirot, N.; Delpech, H.; Broyon, M.; Theillet, C.; Colombo, P.E.; Vie, N.; et al. Anti-tumoral activity of the Pan-HER (Sym013) antibody mixture in gemcitabine-resistant pancreatic cancer models. *Mabs* **2021**, *13*, 1914883. [CrossRef]

32. Marinovic, S.; Berkovic, M.C.; Zjacic-Rotkvic, V.; Kapitanovic, S. Analysis of polymorphisms in EGF, EGFR and *HER2* genes in pancreatic neuroendocrine tumors (PNETs). *Cancer Genet.* **2022**, *266–267*, 44–50. [CrossRef]
33. Ohba, A.; Morizane, C.; Ueno, M.; Kobayashi, S.; Kawamoto, Y.; Komatsu, Y.; Ikeda, M.; Sasaki, M.; Okano, N.; Furuse, J.; et al. Multicenter phase II trial of trastuzumab deruxtecan for *HER2*-positive unresectable or recurrent biliary tract cancer: HERB trial. *Future Oncol.* **2022**, *18*, 2351–2360. [CrossRef] [PubMed]
34. de Vries, E.G.E.; Rüschoff, J.; Lolkema, M.; Tabernero, J.; Gianni, L.; Voest, E.; de Groot, D.J.; Castellano, D.; Erb, G.; Naab, J.; et al. Phase II study (KAMELEON) of single-agent T-DM1 in patients with *HER2*-positive advanced urothelial bladder cancer or pancreatic cancer/cholangiocarcinoma. *Cancer Med.* **2023**, *12*, 12071–12083. [CrossRef] [PubMed]
35. Chou, A.; Waddell, N.; Cowley, M.J.; Gill, A.J.; Chang, D.K.; Patch, A.M.; Nones, K.; Wu, J.; Pinese, M.; Johns, A.L.; et al. Clinical and molecular characterization of *HER2* amplified-pancreatic cancer. *Genome Med.* **2013**, *5*, 78. [CrossRef] [PubMed]
36. Rahib, L.; Smith, B.D.; Aizenberg, R.; Rosenzweig, A.B.; Fleshman, J.M.; Matrisian, L.M. Projecting cancer incidence and deaths to 2030: The unexpected burden of thyroid, liver, and pancreas cancers in the United States. *Cancer Res.* **2014**, *74*, 2913–2921. [CrossRef]
37. Adel, N. Current treatment landscape and emerging therapies for pancreatic cancer. *Am. J. Manag. Care* **2019**, *25*, 3–10.
38. Harder, J.; Ihorst, G.; Heinemann, V.; Hofheinz, R.; Moehler, M.; Buechler, P.; Kloeppel, G.; Röcken, C.; Bitzer, M.; Boeck, S.; et al. Multicentre phase II trial of trastuzumab and capecitabine in patients with *HER2* overexpressing metastatic pancreatic cancer. *Br. J. Cancer* **2012**, *106*, 1033–1038. [CrossRef] [PubMed]
39. Wiggers, J.K.; Ruys, A.T.; Groot Koerkamp, B.; Beuers, U.; ten Kate, F.J.; van Gulik, T.M. Differences in immunohistochemical biomarkers between intra- and extrahepatic cholangiocarcinoma: A systematic review and meta-analysis. *J. Gastroenterol. Hepatol.* **2014**, *29*, 1582–1594. [CrossRef]
40. Tsiambas, E.; Karameris, A.; Dervenis, C.; Lazaris, A.C.; Giannakou, N.; Gerontopoulos, K.; Patsouris, E. *HER2*/neu expression and gene alterations in pancreatic ductal adenocarcinoma: A comparative immunohistochemistry and chromogenic in situ hybridization study based on tissue microarrays and computerized image analysis. *JOP* **2006**, *7*, 283–294.
41. Wood, E.R.; Truesdale, A.T.; McDonald, O.B.; Yuan, D.; Hassell, A.; Dickerson, S.H.; Ellis, B.; Pennisi, C.; Horne, E.; Lackey, K.; et al. A unique structure for epidermal growth factor receptor bound to GW572016 (Lapatinib): Relationships among protein conformation, inhibitor off-rate, and receptor activity in tumor cells. *Cancer Res.* **2004**, *64*, 6652–6659. [CrossRef]
42. Tsurutani, J.; Iwata, H.; Krop, I.; Jänne, P.A.; Doi, T.; Takahashi, S.; Park, H.; Redfern, C.; Tamura, K.; Wise-Draper, T.M.; et al. Targeting *HER2* with trastuzumab deruxtecan: A dose-expansion, phase I study in multiple advanced solid tumors. *Cancer Discov.* **2020**, *10*, 688–701. [CrossRef] [PubMed]
43. Pelzer, U.; Opitz, B.; Deutschinoff, G.; Stauch, M.; Reitzig, P.C.; Hahnfeld, S.; Müller, L.; Grunewald, M.; Stieler, J.M.; Sinn, M.; et al. Efficacy of prophylactic low-molecular weight heparin for ambulatory patients with advanced pancreatic cancer: Outcomes from the CONKO-004 trial. *J. Clin. Oncol.* **2015**, *33*, 2028–2034. [CrossRef] [PubMed]
44. Valsecchi, M.E.; McDonald, M.; Brody, J.R.; Hyslop, T.; Freydin, B.; Yeo, C.J.; Solomides, C.; Peiper, S.C.; Witkiewicz, A.K. Epidermal growth factor receptor and insulinlike growth factor 1 receptor expression predict poor survival in pancreatic ductal adenocarcinoma. *Cancer* **2012**, *118*, 3484–3493. [CrossRef] [PubMed]
45. Pryczynicz, A.; Guzińska-Ustymowicz, K.; Czyzewska, J.; Kemona, A. Expression of epidermal growth factors and apoptosis markers in pancreatic ductal adenocarcinoma. *Folia Histochem. Cytobiol.* **2009**, *47*, 667–671. [CrossRef] [PubMed]
46. Cardin, D.B.; Goff, L.W.; Chan, E.; Whisenant, J.G.; Dan Ayers, G.; Takebe, N.; Arlinghaus, L.R.; Yankeelov, T.E.; Berlin, J.; Merchant, N. Dual Src and EGFR inhibition in combination with gemcitabine in advanced pancreatic cancer: Phase I results: A phase I clinical trial. *Investig. New. Drugs* **2018**, *36*, 442–450. [CrossRef]
47. Nagarkar, R.; Patil, D.; Limaye, S.; Devhare, P.; Ghaisas, A.; Srivastava, N.; Apurwa, S.; Patil, S.; John, J.; Raazi, Z.; et al. Liquid biopsy and multi-analyte testing guided treatment of *HER2* positive periampullary adenocarcinoma with durable complete response after trastuzumab based therapy. *Oncotarget* **2020**, *11*, 4195–4200. [CrossRef]

Journal of Personalized Medicine

MDPI

Systematic Review

Which Is the Best Way to Treat Massive Hemoptysis? A Systematic Review and Meta-Analysis of Observational Studies

Eleni Karlafti [1,2,*], Dimitrios Tsavdaris [3], Evangelia Kotzakioulafi [2], Leonidas Kougias [4], Georgios Tagarakis [5], Georgia Kaiafa [2], Smaro Netta [3], Christos Savopoulos [2], Antonios Michalopoulos [3] and Daniel Paramythiotis [3]

1 Emergency Department, University General Hospital of Thessaloniki AHEPA, Aristotle University of Thessaloniki, 54636 Thessaloniki, Greece
2 1st Propaedeutic Department of Internal Medicine, University General Hospital of Thessaloniki AHEPA, Aristotle University of Thessaloniki, 54636 Thessaloniki, Greece; ekotzaki@auth.gr (E.K.); gdkaiafa@auth.gr (G.K.); csavvopo@auth.gr (C.S.)
3 1st Propaedeutic Surgery Department, University General Hospital of Thessaloniki AHEPA, Aristotle University of Thessaloniki, 54636 Thessaloniki, Greece; tsavdaris@auth.gr (D.T.); smaronetta2@gmail.com (S.N.); amichal@auth.gr (A.M.); danosprx@auth.gr (D.P.)
4 Department of Radiology, University General Hospital of Thessaloniki AHEPA, Aristotle University of Thessaloniki, 54636 Thessaloniki, Greece; leonidaskougias@gmail.com
5 Department of Cardiothoracic Surgery, University General Hospital of Thessaloniki AHEPA, Aristotle University of Thessaloniki, 54636 Thessaloniki, Greece; gtagarakis@auth.gr
* Correspondence: linakarlafti@hotmail.com

Abstract: Introduction: Hemoptysis is one of the most common symptoms of respiratory system diseases. Common causes include bronchiectasis, tumors, tuberculosis, aspergilloma, and cystic fibrosis. The severity of hemoptysis varies from mild to moderate to massive hemoptysis and can easily lead to hemodynamic instability and death from suffocation or shock. Nevertheless, the most threatening hemoptysis that is presented to the emergency department and requires hospitalization is the massive one. In these cases, today, the most common way to manage hemoptysis is bronchial artery embolization (BAE). Methods: A systematic literature search was conducted in PubMed and Scopus from January 2017 (with the aim of selecting the newest possible reports in the literature) until May 2023 for studies reporting massive hemoptysis. All studies that included technical and clinical success rates of hemoptysis management, as well as rebleeding and mortality rates, were included. A proportional meta-analysis was conducted using a random-effects model. Results: Of the 30 studies included in this systematic review, 26 used bronchial artery embolization as a means of treating hemoptysis, with very high levels of both technical and clinical success (greater than 73.7% and 84.2%, respectively). However, in cases where it was not possible to use bronchial artery embolization, alternative methods were used, such as dual-vessel intervention (80% technical success rate and 66.7% clinical success rate), customized endobronchial silicone blockers (92.3% technical success rate and 92.3% clinical success rate), antifibrinolytic agents (50% clinical success rate), and percutaneous transthoracic embolization (93.1% technical success rate and 88.9% clinical success rate), which all had high success rates apart from antifibrinolytic agents. Of the 2467 patients included in these studies, 341 experienced rebleeding during the follow-up period, while 354 other complications occurred, including chest discomfort, fever, dysphagia, and paresis. A total of 89 patients died after an episode of massive hemoptysis or during the follow-up period. The results of the meta-analysis showed a pooled technical success of bronchial artery embolization equal to 97.22% and a pooled clinical success equal to 92.46%. The pooled recurrence was calculated to be 21.46%, while the mortality was 3.5%. These results confirm the ability of bronchial artery embolization in the treatment of massive hemoptysis but also emphasize the high rate of recurrence following the intervention, as well as the risk of death. Conclusion: In conclusion, massive hemoptysis can be treated with great clinical and technical success using bronchial artery embolization, reducing mortality. Mortality has now been reduced to a small percentage of cases.

Keywords: massive hemoptysis; management; bronchial artery embolization; systematic review; meta-analysis

1. Introduction

Respiratory diseases are among the most common reasons for patients visiting hospitals and emergency rooms. These diseases are most commonly manifested by one or more symptoms: cough, chest pain, shortness of breath, or hemoptysis [1]. Further, the SARS-CoV-2 virus infection that broke out recently and quickly spread in a pandemic appears with these symptoms (most commonly, cough and shortness of breath) [2,3]. Hemoptysis may therefore not be the most common clinical finding in COVID-19 patients [4], but it is an urgent situation that requires observation, finding the cause, and taking steps to prevent a more severe recurrence.

Hemoptysis is defined as the expulsion of blood through the oral tract from a source located in the lower respiratory tract, i.e., below the level of the glottis [5,6]. It is a frequent clinical finding that is usually due to bronchitis, pneumonia, bronchiectasis, tuberculosis, neoplasms (bronchial carcinoma, intrabronchial tumors, sarcomas, and metastases), or even pulmonary embolism [5–10]. Other less common causes include coagulopathy, platelet disorders, pulmonary hypertension, aneurysm rupture, trauma (catheter, biopsy, iatrogenic, or blunt trauma), foreign body aspiration, vascular and collagen diseases (such as Goodpasture's syndrome, Behçet's disease, systemic lupus erythematosus, granulomatosis with polyangiitis, Henoch–Schonlein purpura, and rheumatoid arthritis), drugs and narcotics (such as anticoagulants, penicillamine, solvents, crack, and cocaine), and even gastric content aspiration or cryptogenic causes [5–12]. Its extent can vary from the presence of blood in the sputum to potentially life-threatening massive hemoptysis [8]. The etiology of hemoptysis affects the choice of appropriate treatment [5,6,9,11].

Massive hemoptysis is defined as blood loss that exceeds 600 mL per twenty-four hours or 150 mL per hour [8]. Massive hemoptysis is related to pathologies that alter the pulmonary vasculature, usually affecting the bronchial arteries, and can be either inflammatory or neoplastic. This emergency can easily and quickly lead to death due to airway obstruction and hypoxemia from asphyxiation, rather than hemodynamic disturbance and shock, which do not occur early [9]. Even a tiny vessel rupture can have significant clinical consequences because of aspiration and the difficulty of stable thrombus formation that prevents vessel healing in thin-walled airways. Due to the severity of the situation, it is necessary to differentiate between the conditions with a similar picture which are characterized as pseudohemoptysis [13]. These can be upper digestive, upper respiratory, or even oral cavity bleeding. Hemoptysis has a bright red color as well as an alkaline frothy sputum, while in other cases of pseudohemoptysis the blood is acidic and darker in color [10,13].

Two pathways are blamed as pathophysiological mechanisms. The first and most common one concerns bleeding from the bronchial arteries because they handle higher pressures [10,14–17]. This pathway begins when diseases cause hypoxic vasospasm and thereby limit pulmonary circulation. This implies an increase in blood supply with an increase in the rupture of the fragile anastomotic vessels and bleeding into the alveoli and bronchi. Other causative diseases are those that, through the release of angiogenic growth factors, cause neovascularization and the development of collateral circulation. These vessels are also fragile, and so their rupture causes hemoptysis. Hemoptysis, however, can also occur from the vessels of the pulmonary circulation, either iatrogenically during catheterization, during aneurysm rupture, or from other causes [10,14–17].

According to the guidelines [5,9–11,18], the first step is to diagnose massive hemoptysis. The diagnostic algorithm includes a general blood test as well as a coagulation profile. The imaging examination usually does not start with an X-ray because the diagnostic accuracy and detection of bleeding are poor. For this reason, other imaging tests are preferred.

These include bronchoscopy, which can detect bleeding in over 90% of cases. Another advantage of this examination is that it does not require moving the patient, while at the same time it offers information about the patient's anatomy, a fact that facilitates subsequent intervention, increasing its effectiveness [19–21]. An alternative method is computed tomography (CT), which has been shown to be even more effective in detecting bleeding and can therefore replace bronchoscopy. Although it is an unusual finding, bronchial artery bleeding can be seen at the time of the scan. This can indicate the site and cause of the bleeding. Native CT can also indicate the site of bleeding, which may manifest as a ground glass infiltration or as pulmonary consolidation, and permit the identification of the site of major architectural distortion in the case of diffuse pathologies [22]. CT angiography permits the identification of the origin of bronchial arteries from the thoracic aorta and facilitates catheterization during interventional angiography. A bronchial artery diameter greater than 3 mm is usually considered pathologic. There is great variability in the number and site of origin of the bronchial arteries, but the most usual patterns are one or two arteries for each lung that originate from the descending thoracic aorta around the level of the tracheal bifurcation. Sometimes, a bronchial artery may arise as a common trunk with an intercostal artery. On the other hand, lung pathology located superficially may result in neovascularization from intercostal artery branches or from internal mammary arteries [5,9,10,16,23–25].

Then, according to the guidelines, the hemoptysis is treated [26–28]. The treatment of massive hemoptysis has two aspects. The first concerns the emergency arrest of bleeding which does not stop spontaneously and constitutes an emergency. This can be accomplished by using a rigid bronchoscope and adequate aspiration of blood, as well as intubation of the lung and occlusion of the bleeding site, e.g., with a balloon, to ensure a non-bleeding lung. Finally, hemostatic drugs, such as pituitrin, hemocoagulase, and others such as carbazochrome sulfonate sodium and carbazochrome tablets, are applied. Therefore, after the diagnosis is made and emergency treatment is applied, where necessary, follow-up targeted treatment of massive hemoptysis is required. In this phase, the main technique used is bronchial artery embolization (BAE). Alternatives are surgical treatment of the bleeding or etiological treatment [5,9–11,18]. The prognosis of massive hemoptysis is indicated by several factors. These include the amount of blood in the sputum, the etiology of hemoptysis (such as cancer), and hemodynamic instability [29,30].

Furthermore, for the treatment of massive hemoptysis, it is important to take certain factors into serious consideration. These include coagulation parameters as well as the taking of anticoagulant drugs. Specifically, the number of platelets determines the safety of both biopsy (safety thresholds of more than 50,000/mm^3) and bronchoscopy (safety thresholds of more than 20,000/mm^3) [31,32]. Anticoagulation, especially colpidogrel, also increases the risk of bleeding during procedures such as biopsies [33]. From the laboratory findings, urea and BUN are also considered important, as uremia and BUN > 30 mg/dL increase the risk of bleeding during surgery [34].

Since massive hemoptysis is a life-threatening condition, an effective treatment method is essential. Massive hemoptysis, unlike mild hemoptysis, is primarily treated invasively. BAE is considered the method of choice and the first in line. This method can be applied with various techniques. One of the most common is the Seldinger technique. The Seldinger technique usually uses the right femoral artery for access and selective catheterization of the bronchial and intercostal arteries using a 5 French catheter (Cobra, Simmons or DESLER), which is inserted through the diagnostic catheter a few centimeters distally to the vessel origin. This setup provides stability and impedes reflux of embolic material to the thoracic aorta or into radiculomedullary vessels, which, when present, arise as proximal branches [35–37]. Catheterization of bronchial arteries and contrast injection will demonstrate enlarged, tortuous vessels with intense angiographic blush in the parenchymal phase of the angiography. This pathologic imaging pattern is enough to justify embolization, given that active contrast extravasation is usually not observed. Each angiographic run should also be thoroughly examined to identify possible branches directed to the spinal canal. Sometimes, radiculomedullary arteries may arise from bronchial arteries as anatomic variations or from a costobronchial trunk. The dominant radiculomedullary artery is the artery of Adamkievitch and provides a major contribution to the anterior spinal artery. This branch presents a characteristic hairpin configuration and projects on the vertebral column along the midline. If angiographic interpretation is difficult, rotational angiography with 3D reconstructions might help. Superselective catheterization of anomalous arteries using 2-F microcatheters is chosen, where possible, for the best results. Several different techniques for access and embolization may be used as appropriate. Also, embolic agents, such as polyvinyl alcohol, coils, gelatin sponges, and Embospheres, are more common [35–37]. The embolic materials of choice are particles or microspheres. They should not be smaller than 250 microns, otherwise the probability of their entering dangerous collaterals, leading to non-target embolization, is increased. Coils should be avoided because a new embolization session in case of a relapse will be impossible [17]. It is important to identify and embolize the bronchial artery that supplies the responsible pulmonary lobe, but in cases of diffuse pathologies, embolization of all identified pathologic vessels can be considered, case by case, to prevent future bleeding episodes. The double vascularization of the pulmonary parenchyma usually prevents ischemic complications.

Therefore, knowledge regarding the treatment of massive hemoptysis is necessary to reduce mortality risk. This systematic review aims to evaluate the available treatments for massive hemoptysis according to the latest available studies in the literature, including evaluation of the technical and clinical success of the methods for managing hemoptysis, as well as recurrence, complications, and mortality. The technical success of an operation is defined as successful intervention in massive hemoptysis, i.e., successful bronchial embolization of the bleeding arteries and arrest of the bleeding. Clinical success is defined as the resolution of the clinical findings of massive hemoptysis after the application of the intervention, that is, the cessation of hemoptysis and other clinical findings that the patient may present.

2. Materials and Methods

2.1. Study Protocol and Guidelines

This systematic review was written according to the Preferred Reporting Items for Systematic Reviews and Meta-Analyses (PRISMA) guidelines [38]. This systematic review is registered in the Open Science Framework (OSF) with the registration number: DOI osf.io/r2n8w.

2.2. Eligibility Criteria

The eligibility criteria for this systematic review are presented and were defined with the PICO framework. To be included in this systematic review, studies had to meet the following inclusion criteria:

1. Involve adult patients with massive hemoptysis;
2. Report on the management of massive hemoptysis;
3. Provide technical and clinical success rates of the treatment used;
4. Include data on recurrence and mortality.

Reviews, letters, comments, and case reports were excluded. Only original articles that met the above criteria were included.

2.3. Information Sources, Search Strategy, and Selection Process

A systematic literature search was conducted in two databases (PubMed and Scopus) using the keywords 'massive hemoptysis' and 'management'. The search was limited to a six-year period from January 2017 (with the aim of selecting the newest possible studies in the literature) until May 2023 and articles had to be written in English to be selected. The selection process was carried out by two independent reviewers (D.T. and E. Kar.) using Rayyan [39], who assessed the studies for inclusion in this systematic review. The two reviewers were blinded during both the title and abstract screening and the full-text screening. Any disagreement was resolved by a third reviewer (E. Kot.).

2.4. Data Collection Process and Data Items

Data extraction was carried out by one reviewer (D.T.), and another reviewer (E.Kot.) independently checked the results. The data were extracted in a standardized Excel form. Data extraction was performed without the use of any automation tools. From the studies that were reviewed, the relevant data for extraction were: the main characteristics of each study; the identity of each study (author and year of publication); the total number of participants, along with the mean age and the percentage of men; the type of study; the management of bleeding; and the technical success rate of the method used.

2.5. Quality Assessment

Quality assessment of the included studies was performed using the Newcastle–Ottawa Quality Assessment Scale for Cohort Studies by two independent reviewers (D.T. and E.Kar.). Any disagreement was resolved by a third reviewer (E.Kot.). The Newcastle–Ottawa tool consists of three evaluation domains. These are the selection of the participating patients, comparability, and outcomes. The selection of participants includes: the representativeness of the exposed cohort, the selection of the non-exposed cohort, the ascertainment of exposure, and a demonstration that the outcome of interest was not present at the start of the study. With respect to the first question regarding the representativeness of the exposed cohort, a star is given when the sample is truly or somewhat representative. Regarding the selection of the non-exposed cohort, a star is given if the selection of the non-exposed cohort is drawn from the same community as the exposed cohort. To be given a star for the ascertainment of exposure, a secure record or structured interviews must be presented. Finally, the last star is given if there is a demonstration that the outcome of interest was not present at the start of the study. Regarding the 2nd domain, on comparability, two stars may be given for the comparability of cohorts if the design or analysis controlled for confounders. For the outcomes, the assessment of outcomes and the follow-ups are evaluated. For the first, a star is given if the assessment was independent and blind or a record linkage, while for the follow-up, a star is given if the assessment was sufficient to evaluate the results and if several of the participants were included in it.

2.6. Statistical Analysis

Statistical analysis was conducted with R studio (R Core Team (2022). R: A language and environment for statistical computing. R Foundation for Statistical Computing, Vienna, Austria. URL: https://www.R-project.org/ (accessed on 8 September 2023)). A proportional meta-analysis was conducted using the metafor [40] and meta packages [41] using a random-effects model. Cases and total numbers of participants were extracted for each outcome from each individual study, and their proportions were calculated during the meta-analysis. Publication bias was determined with visual inspection of funnel plots for each outcome and Egger's test [42]. Heterogeneity is presented with I^2 results, and results between 0 and 40% were considered instances of non-important heterogeneity, those between 40 and 60% instances of moderate heterogeneity, those between 60 and 75% instances of substantial heterogeneity, and those between 75 and 100% instances of considerable heterogeneity [43,44].

3. Results

3.1. Study Selection

A total of 785 studies were found using the keywords 'treatment' and 'massive hemoptysis', 395 of them in PubMed and 390 in Scopus. Of these, 658 were excluded, as they were either duplicates or letters, case reports, reviews, or comments. Thus, the remaining 127 studies were screened for eligibility, 30 of which met the inclusion criteria and were assessed for eligibility in the full-text screening. These studies therefore analyzed the success rate of the management of massive hemoptysis. The screening process for the studies selected for inclusion in this systematic review is illustrated in a PRISMA 2020 flow chart (Figure 1). All selection stages from the initial stage to the final stage are depicted.

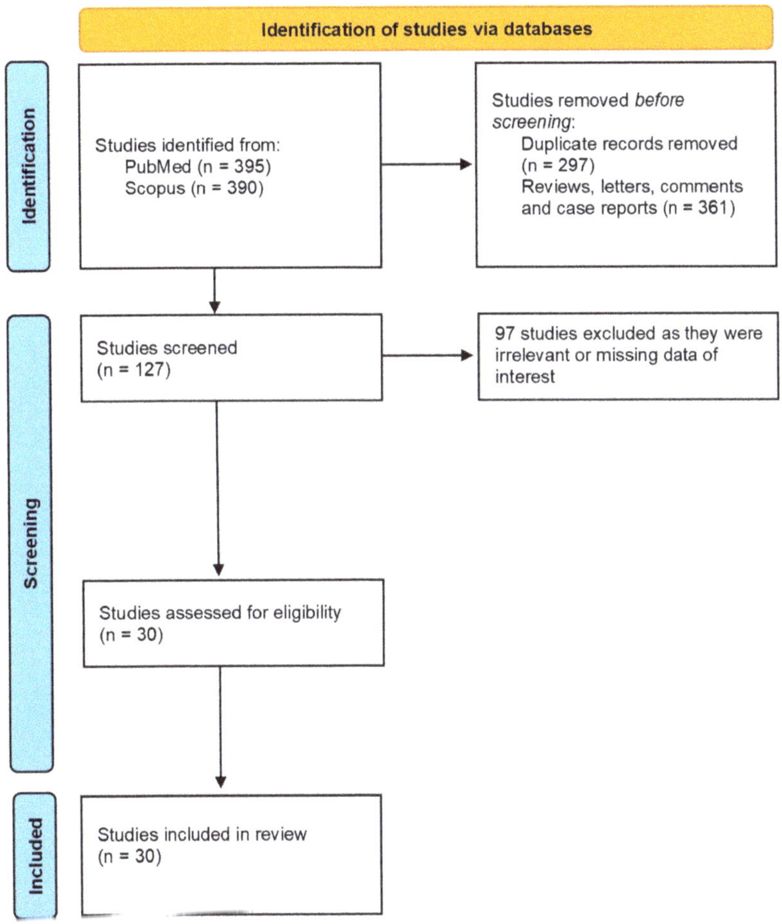

Figure 1. PRISMA 2020 flow chart. This diagram illustrates the process followed for the collection and selection of studies used in our systematic review.

3.2. Study Characteristics

3.2.1. Major Characteristics of the Included Studies

The 30 studies included 2647 patients who developed massive hemoptysis and were treated accordingly [45–74]. In these studies, treatment was applied either to stop bleeding in cases of massive hemoptysis in which conservative treatment was unsuccessful or to prevent recurrent bleeding. All these studies were retrospective observational cohort studies. The largest sample size was 489 patients, in Ishikawa et al., 2017 [49]. This study was conducted in Japan by a center specializing in hemoptysis. In contrast, the smallest sample size was found in Clements et al., 2022 [72], with only three patients. Finally, the majority of studies (26/30) used bronchial artery embolization for managing massive hemoptysis. Despite the common methods applied in all these investigations, the different tools, materials, and techniques applied in each investigation are of interest. These are presented in Table 1.

Table 1. Characteristics of included studies.

Study ID	Total Subjects (% Male/ Median Age)	Study Type	Management of Hemoptysis	Technical Success Rate	Clinical Success Rate
Abid et al., 2021 [74]	46 (78.2/54.8)	ORCS	BAE	97.5	95
Yang et al., 2022 [73]	15 (80/55.9)	ORCS	Dual-vessel intervention	80	66.7
Clements et al., 2022 [72]	3	ORCS	BAE	100	100
Mishra et al., 2018 [71]	52 (82.6/48)	ORCS	BAE	NM	92
Silveira et al., 2021 [70]	17 (47/25)	ORCS	BAE	100	NM
Seyyedi et al., 2019 [69]	189 (58.3/NM)	ORCS	BAE	NM	97.3
Fu et al., 2019 [68]	24	ORCS	BAE	94.9	91.7
Ando et al., 2017 [67]	35	ORCS	BAE	94.3	97
Kolu et et al., 2022 [66]	48 (68.7/52)	ORCS	BAE	97.9	93.7
Mehta et al., 2020 [65]	12	ORCS	Customized endobronchial silicone blocker	92.3	92.3
Keshmiri et al., 2020 [64]	153 (68/55)	ORCS	BAE	100	NM
Marcelin et al., 2018 [63]	19 (78.9/60.3)	ORCS	BAE	73.7	84.2
Miyano et al., 2017 [62]	179	ORCS	BAE	93.2	92.8
Xiaobing et al., 2022 [61]	187	ORCS	BAE	100	86.6
Han et al., 2019 [60]	84	ORCS	BAE	98.9	82.1
Seki et al., 2017 [59]	10	ORCS	BAE	100	100
Al-Samkari et al., 2019 [58]	21	ORCS	Antifibrinolytic agents	NM	50
Floridi et al., 2022 [57]	13 (NM/NM)	ORCS	BAE	94.7	92.3
Kucukay et al., 2018 [56]	174 (45.9/39.4)	ORCS	BAE	100	91.9
Lal et al., 2021 [55]	27 (NM/ 41.4)	ORCS	Percutaneous transthoracic embolisation	93.1	88.9
Lee et al., 2022 [54]	19	ORCS	BAE	94.7	89.5
Frood et al., 2020 [53]	68 (60.2/53)	ORCS	BAE	90	86.5
Flight et al., 2017 [52]	27	ORCS	BAE		
Springer et al., 2018 [51]	30 (NM/33.5)	ORCS	BAE	NM	95.75
Le-Jun et al., 2020 [50]	5	ORCS	BAE	100	100
Ishikawa et al., 2017 [49]	489 (46.4/69)	ORCS	BAE	93.4	92
Ando et al., 2019 [48]	41	ORCS	BAE	NM	92.7
An et al., 2023 [47]	17	ORCS	BAE	100	100
Li et al., 2023 [46]	105 (64/NM)	ORCS	BAE	NM	84.8
Cheng et al., 2023 [45]	127 (Group E: 47/58, Group G: 53/60)	ORCS	BAE using Embospheres alone and Embospheres with gelfoam particles	92.99 & 97.14	85.96 & 97.14

Abbreviations: ORCS: observational retrospective cohort study, BAE: bronchial artery embolization.

3.2.2. Findings of the Studies

Some studies used techniques that differed greatly or slightly from bronchial artery embolization or used the classical technique of bronchial artery embolization with various variations depending on the circumstances and characteristics of the patients. Kucukay et al. [56] used large-sized (700–900 lm) tris-acryl microspheres (Embospheres) for bronchial embolization. The results showed the great clinical success of this technique, with very high long-term success rates. Specifically, clinical success reached 100%. The disadvantage of this technique is that the microspheres, due to their large size, can occlude the bronchial artery, which is much more central to the lesion. However, the use of a microcatheter significantly reduces the likelihood of this happening.

Xiaobing et al. and Seki et al. [59,61] used chemotherapeutic substances as means of embolization of the coronary arteries. This variant is called bronchial artery chemoembolization and seems to be advantageous over the classic technique with respect to the long-term results of treating hemoptysis due to lung cancer. It requires repeated courses of treatment, and various substances, such as epirubicin, nedaplatin, and etoposide, are used. The trophic arteries of the tumor are embolized, and it seems to be a technique that solves the problem of the difficult management of hemoptysis in cancer patients. This difficulty is due to the different and complex pathophysiology of hemoptysis in lung cancer. BAE, on the other hand, does not manage the tumor but only the hemoptysis, leading to the high recurrence rates in these patients.

In cases of anomalies, such as pseudoaneurysms, Marcelin et al. [63] suggested the use of pulmonary embolization versus bronchial embolization or endoprosthesis placement. This technique scored a high success rate relative to the difficulty and severity of the condition, while two patients died due to massive bleeding. The stent ensures the patency of the vessel; however, a complication is its occlusion due to the stent.

Mehta et al. [65] evaluated the use of customized endobronchial silicone blockers for the management of massive hemoptysis in cases where BAE is not an option. With this technique, a customized endobronchial silicone blocker is used to wedge and occlude the bleeding, with quite favourable results. The clinical success rate reached 92.3%, making this technique successful enough to replace BAE where it is not possible. Its only flaw is that it has not been studied as well as BAE to ensure its safety and success. Yang et al. [73] used the dual-vessel intervention (DVI) technique. This is a less successful technique that scored technical and clinical rates of 80% and 66.7%, respectively. This technique includes bronchial and pulmonary artery embolization with a hyperselective catheter and the use of PVA and a spring coil. Finally, the lowest clinical success rate was achieved in Samkari et al. [58], who used antifibrinolytic agents to manage hemoptysis. However, this percentage was also affected by the population group, as it included patients with cystic fibrosis, who have high failure rates in operations.

An et al. [47] examined bronchial artery embolization with a specific opening, namely, the opening of the lower wall of the aortic arch. This study reports that this method was particularly effective, with fewer complications and rebleeding, and involved the use of the JL4 catheter. The use of this catheter is particularly important, as operations of this type have not been as successful as operations using other catheters. The advantages of this catheter are found in its shape, its rigidity, and the absence of the need to create a loop.

Finally, Cheng et al. [45] analyzed the safety and effectiveness of the use of embospheres alone or in combination with gelfoam particles for BAE. The results showed that the combination of these gave significantly better results, with technical and clinical success scores of 97.14% and 97.14%, respectively. The use of pure embospheres scored technical and clinical success rates of 92.99% and 85.96%, respectively. Therefore, the major difference between these two is found in the clinical success of the two techniques. For this reason, the authors suggest the use of embospheres together with gelfoam particles to avoid clinical failure.

Etiology of Massive Hemoptysis

In the studies included in this systematic review, bronchiectasis is reported as the first cause, in 658 reported cases out of 2647 in total, thus covering a quarter of the causes of massive bleeding (Table 2 and Figure 2). This is followed by tumors and tuberculosis, comprising 444 and 397 cases, respectively. Cases of aspergilloma and cystic fibrosis are also common and require special management.

Table 2. Etiology of massive hemoptysis in the studies included in this systematic review.

Etiology of Massive Hemoptysis	Number of Incidents
Bronchiectasis	658
Tumor	444
Tuberculosis	397
Cystic fibrosis	64
Pulmonary artery pseudoaneurysms	29
Aspergilloma	196

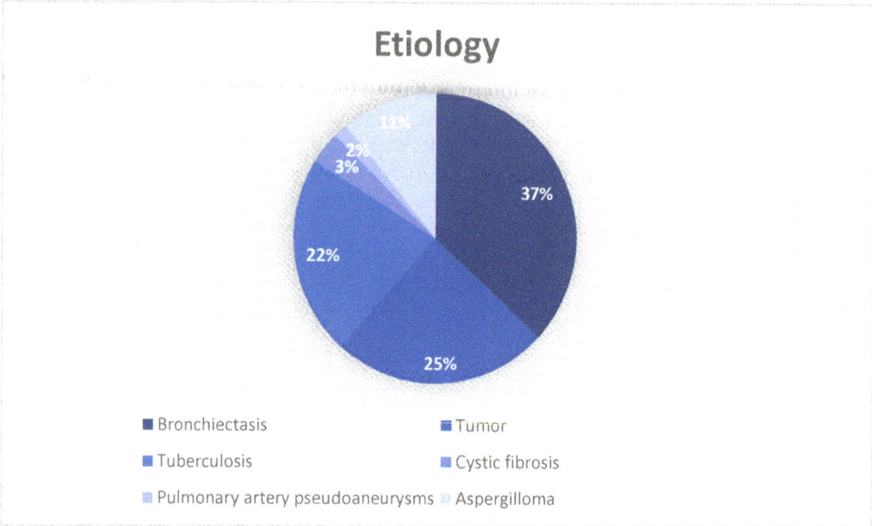

Figure 2. Etiology of massive hemoptysis.

Radiological and Angiographic Findings

In the studies included in this systematic review, 460 cases of hypertrophy and dilatation, 44 cases of parenchymal hypervascularity, 145 cases of parenchymal blush, 73 cystic findings, 37 cavities, and 78 aneurysms were reported (Table 3). However, these numbers underestimate the actual findings because many of the studies did not report the number of findings included in the overall result.

Table 3. Radiological and angiographic findings.

Angiographic Findings	Incidence
Hypertrophy and dilatation	460
Parenchymal hypervascularity	44
Parenchymatous blush	145
Cystic lesion	73
Cavity	37
Aneurysmal lesion	78

Recurrence, Complications, and Mortality

Table 4 presents the main postoperative complications, rebleedings, and deaths that were recorded. The main complication was chest pain, sometimes mild and sometimes more severe, which required investigation and treatment with analgesics. At least 140 such cases were reported in the studies included in this systematic review. The next most-frequent complication was fever (52 cases reported), but no further details were available from the studies regarding its cause. Only 11 cases of dysphagia and throat discomfort were reported, while even fewer, i.e., 2, were cases of paresis, one of the serious complications of the operation. A total of 149 more complications were reported, including nausea/vomiting (the most common), headache, and abdominal pain, while some of the serious and life-threatening complications reported were aortic dissection, cerebellar infarctions, and hematomas.

Table 4. Recurrence, complications, and mortality.

Study ID	Chest Discomfort	Fever	Dysphagia and Throat Discomfort	Paresis	Other Complications	Recurrence	Mortality
Abid et al., 2021 [74]	2	0	0	0	1 (headache)	6/46	1
Yang et al., 2022 [73]	6	0	0	0	12 (ventricular arrhythmia)	2/15	1
Clements et al., 2022 [72]	0	0	0	0	0	0/3	0
Mishra et al., 2018 [71]	5	0	0	1	0	2/52	1
Silveira et al., 2021 [70]	0	0	0	0	0	10/17	3
Seyyedi et al., 2019 [69]	23	0	10	0	6 (subintimal dissection, and pancreatitis)	53/189	20
Fu et al., 2019 [68]	6	2	0	0	1 (vagus reflex)	2/207	0
Ando et al., 2017 [67]	12	0	0	0	0	10/35	
Kolu et et al., 2022 [66]	5	0	0	0	0	4/45	1
Mehta et al., 2020 [65]	0	0	0	0	0	1/13	0
Keshmiri et al., 2020 [64]	0	0	0	0	3 (ischemia, pulmonary infarction, and spinal complications)	43/153	1
Marcelin et al., 2018 [63]	0	0	0	0	0	0/19	2
Miyano et al., 2017 [62]	0	0	0	0	1 (aortic dissection)	12/179	3
Xiaobing et al., 2022 [61]	34	38	0	0	87 (nausea/vomiting, increase in AST/ALT, decrease in platelets, abdominal pain)	NM	15
Han et al., 2019 [60]	0	0	0	0	0	20/84	2
Seki et al., 2017 [59]	1	0	0	0	1 (allergic reaction)	3/10	2/10
Al-Samkari et al., 2019 [58]	NM	NM	NM	NM	NM	NM	NM
Floridi et al., 2022 [57]	NM	NM	NM	NM	NM	NM	NM
Kucukay et al., 2018 [56]	9	NM	NM	NM	NM	14/174	0
Lal et al., 2021 [55]	0	0	0	0	1 (pneumothorax)	1/29	0
Lee et al., 2022 [54]	0	0	0	0	0	7/19	0
Frood et al., 2020 [53]	0	0	0	1	2 (cardio-pulmonary arrest, cerebellar infarction)	NM	NM
Flight et al., 2017 [52]	14	0	0	0	15 (paraesthesia, headache)	31/49	5
Springer et al., 2018 [51]	0	1	0	0	3 (1 haematoma at the site of microcatheter insertion and 2 vomiting)	10/30	6
Le-Jun et al., 2020 [50]	0	0	0	0	0	0	0
Ishikawa et al., 2017 [49]	NM	NM	NM	NM	8 (1 aortic dissection, 2 symptomatic cerebellar infarctions, and 5 mediastinal haematoma cases)	57/489	23
Ando et al., 2019 [48]	NM	NM	NM	NM	NM	21/41	NM
An et al., 2023 [47]	6	5	1	0	0	3/17	0
Li et al., 2023 [46]	8	1	0	0	1 (nausea)	29/64	NM
Cheng et al., 2023 [45]	9	5	0	0	7 (2 vomiting, 2 poor appetite, 2 allergy, 1 transient cortical blindness)	NM	3
TOTAL	140	52	11	2	149	341/1979	89

Regarding the occurrence of rebleeding, 341 cases occurred out of 1979 cases, while it is not known what happened to the remaining 668 cases due to a lack of data. These cases of rebleeding, however, were recorded at different follow-up times, that is, some appeared in the first month after the operation, others in the first six months, others in the first year, and so on. A total of 89 deaths related to hemoptysis were also recorded, which highlights the seriousness and danger of the condition, as well as the need for proper and effective treatment.

3.3. *Quality Assessment*

The results from the quality assessment using the Newscastle–Ottawa Scale are listed in Table 5. The included studies did not use non-exposed cohorts and were not given a star in the selection domain.

Table 5. Quality assessment of included studies.

Study ID	Selection				Comparability	Outcome			Total	Quality
	Representativeness of the Exposed Cohort	Selection of the Non-Exposed Cohort	Ascertainment of Exposure	Demonstration That Outcome of Interest Was Not Present at Start of Study	Comparability of Cohorts on the Basis of the Design or Analysis Controlled for Confounders	Assessment of Outcome	Follow-Up Long Enough for Outcomes to Occur	Adequacy of Follow-Up of Cohorts		
Yang et al., 2022 [73]	*		*	*	**	*	*	*	8/9	Good
Clements et al., 2022 [72]	*		*	*	**	*	*	*	8/9	Good
Mishra et al., 2018 [71]	*		*	*	**	*	*	*	8/9	Good
Silveira et al., 2021 [70]	*		*	*	**	*	*	*	8/9	Good
Seyyedi et al., 2019 [69]	*		*	*	**	*	*	*	8/9	Good
Fu et al., 2019 [68]	*		*	*	**	*	*	*	8/9	Good
Ando et al., 2017 [67]	*		*	*	**	*	*	*	8/9	Good
Kolu et et al., 2022 [66]	*		*	*	**	*	*	*	8/9	Good
Mehta et al., 2020 [65]	*		*	*	**	*	*	*	8/9	Good
Keshmiri et al., 2020 [64]	*		*	*	**	*	*	*	8/9	Good
Marcelin et al., 2018 [63]	*		*	*	**	*	*	*	8/9	Good
Miyano et al., 2017 [62]	*		*	*	**	*	*	*	8/9	Good
Xiaobing et al., 2022 [61]	*		*	*	**	*	*	*	8/9	Good
Han et al., 2019 [60]	*		*	*	**	*	*	*	8/9	Good
Seki et al., 2017 [59]	*		*	*	**	*	*	*	8/9	Good
Al-Samkari et al., 2019 [58]	*		*	*	**	*	*	*	8/9	Good
Floridi et al., 2022 [57]	*		*	*	**	*	*	*	8/9	Good
Kucukay et al., 2018 [56]	*		*	*	**	*	*	*	8/9	Good
Lal et al., 2021 [55]	*		*	*	**	*	*	*	8/9	Good
Lee et al., 2022 [54]	*		*	*	**	*	*	*	8/9	Good
Frood et al., 2020 [53]	*		*	*	**	*	*	*	8/9	Good
Flight et al., 2017 [52]	*		*	*	**	*	*	*	8/9	Good
Springer et al., 2018 [51]	*		*	*	**	*	*	*	8/9	Good
Le-Jun et al., 2020 [50]	*		*	*	**	*	*	*	8/9	Good
Ishikawa et al., 2017 [49]	*		*	*	**	*	*	*	8/9	Good
Ando et al., 2019 [48]	*		*	*	**	*	*	*	8/9	Good
An et al., 2023 [47]	*		*	*	**	*	*	[illegible]	8/9	Good
Li et al., 2023 [46]	*		*	*	**	*	*	*	8/9	Good
Cheng et al., 2023 [45]	*		*	*	**	*	*	*	8/9	Good
Abid et al., 2021 [74]	*		*	*	**	*	*	*	8/9	Good

With *, the star given to each category that excludes the risk of bias is denoted. Each category is evaluated with a blank or a *, except for the Comparability category which is evaluated with a blank or a * or **.

3.4. Meta-Analysis Results

A proportional meta-analysis was performed for all studies that used a common mode of management of massive hemoptysis, that is, BAE, and provided relevant data [45–54,56,57,59–64,66,68–72,74].

3.4.1. Technical Success Meta-Analysis

The results of the statistical analysis showed a pooled technical success rate of 97.22%, confirming the technical success of the operation. Technical success is defined as successful embolization of the bronchial arteries. These results are presented with a forest plot in Figure 3. Significant heterogeneity between the included studies was observed ($I^2 = 77\%$, $p < 0.001$). Publication bias for technical success presented significant asymmetry (Figure 4, $p = 0.0024$).

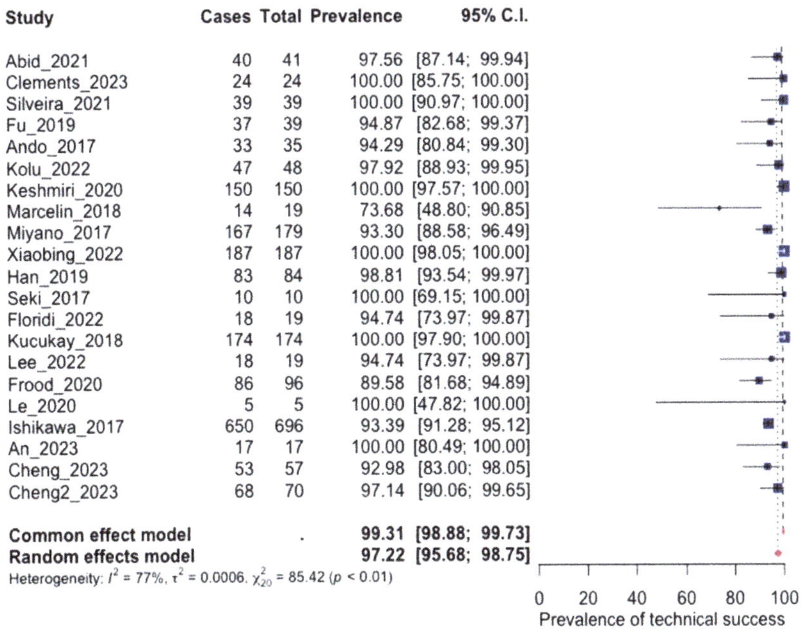

Figure 3. Forest plot for technical success [45,47,49,50,53,54,56,57,59–64,66–68,70,72,74].

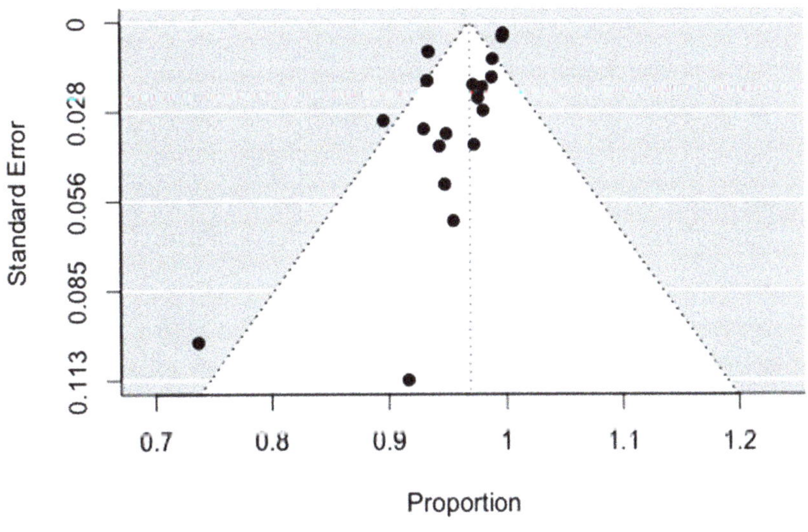

Figure 4. Funnel plot for technical success.

3.4.2. Clinical Success

Clinical success is defined as complete cessation of hemoptysis after bronchial arterial embolization. The statistical analysis of the results of 24 studies showed a pooled clinical success equal to 92.46% (90.43; 94.50 95% CI), with moderate heterogeneity (I^2: 57%, $p < 0.001$). These results confirm the effectiveness of BAE in treating massive hemoptysis. No significant asymmetry was observed in the funnel plot regarding publication bias ($p = 0.0772$). The results are presented in Figures 5 and 6.

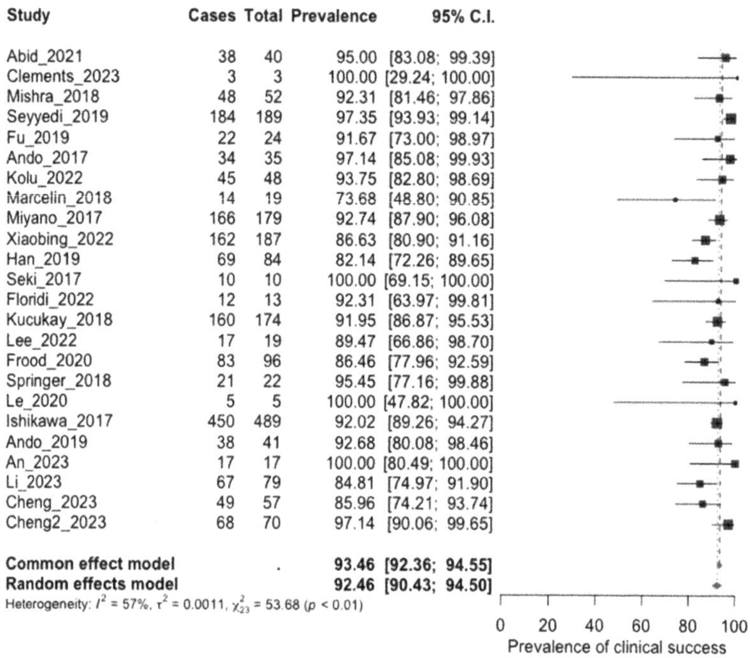

Figure 5. Forest plot for clinical success [45–51,53,54,56,57,59–63,66–69,71,72,74].

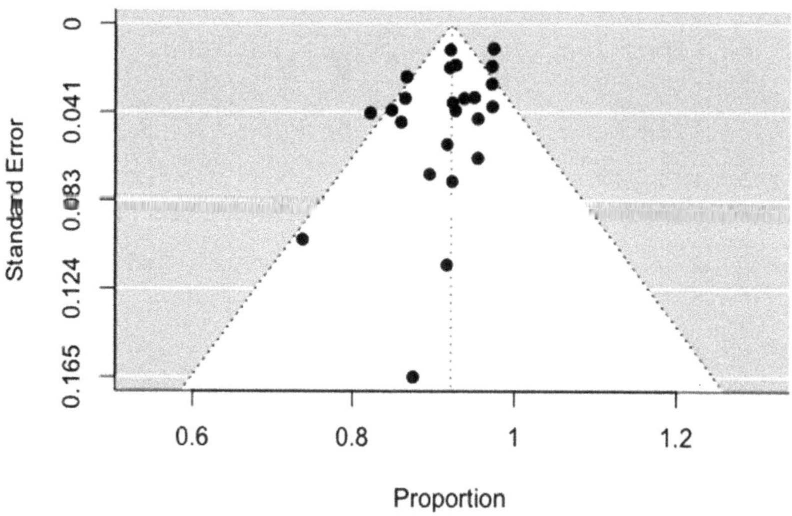

Figure 6. Funnel plot for clinical success.

3.4.3. Recurrence

All episodes of recurrence and rebleeding recorded in the studies in this systematic review during follow-up were used to calculate the prevalence of recurrence. The pooled recurrence was calculated to be equal to 21.46% (14.04; 28.89 95% CI), which shows the frequent occurrence of recurrence in patients, which can often be life-threatening. The result was considered statistically significant, with $p < 0.0001$, while high heterogeneity was also distinguished. These results are visible in Figures 7 and 8, below.

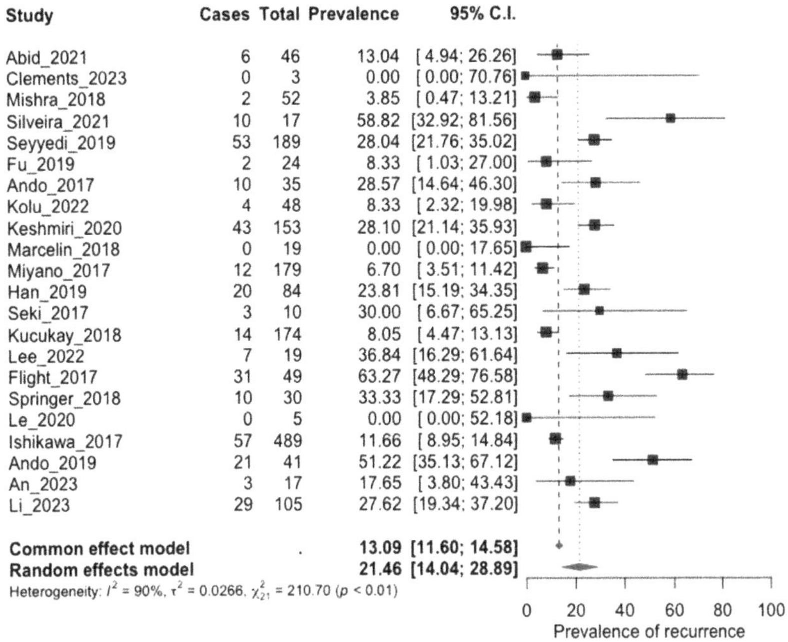

Figure 7. Forest plot for recurrence [46–52,54,56,59,60,62–64,66–72,74].

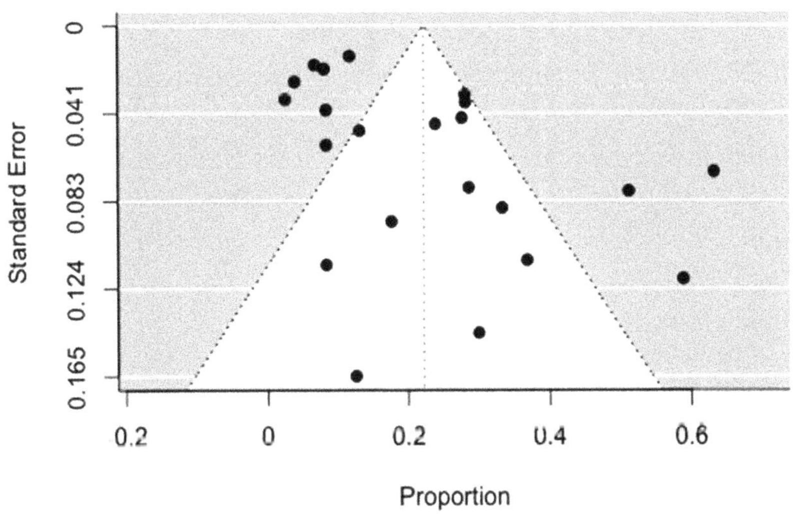

Figure 8. Regression test for funnel plot asymmetry. Significant asymmetry was observed ($p = 0.0246$).

3.4.4. Mortality

The pooled result for mortality was 3.5% (95% CI: 1.78; 5.21). Mortality, although it is a rare complication of massive hemoptysis, is a real risk that has not yet been eliminated. Significant asymmetry was observed in the funnel plot, indicating publication bias (p = 0.0002). The results are presented in Figures 9 and 10.

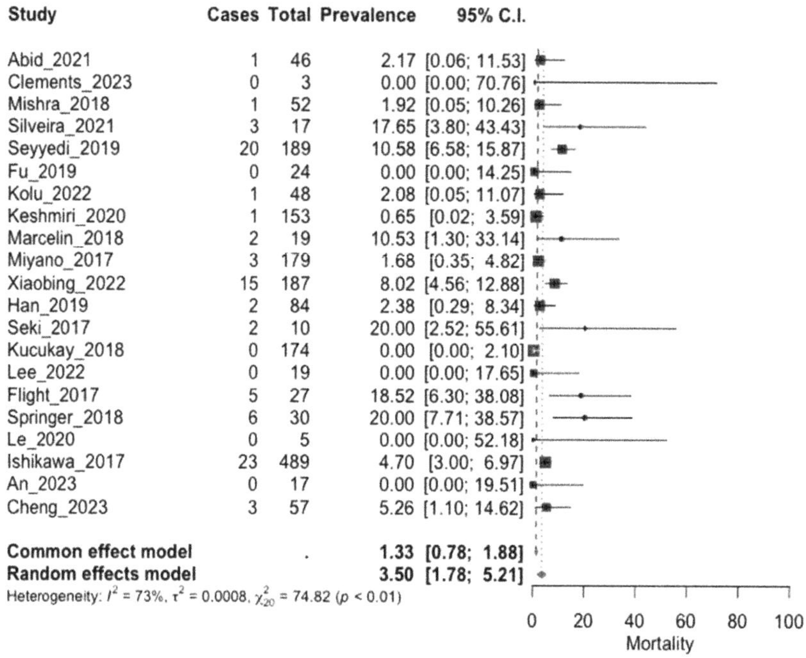

Figure 9. Forest plot for mortality [45,47,49–52,54,56,59–64,66,68–72,74].

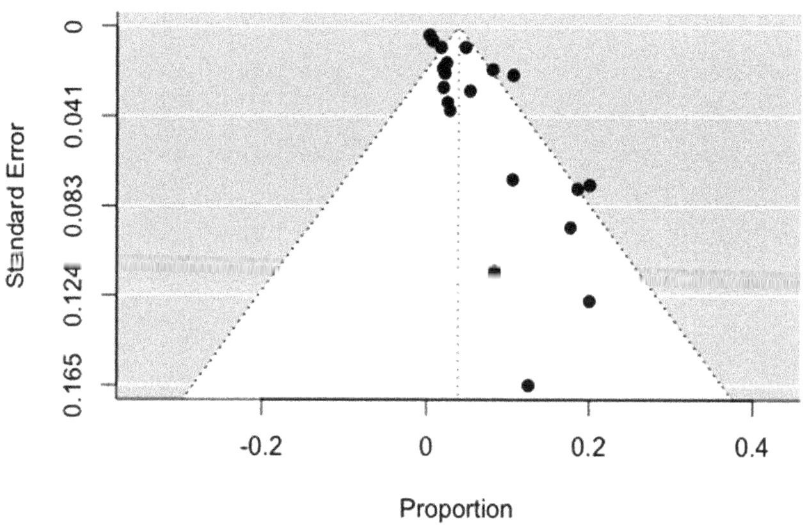

Figure 10. Funnel plot for mortality.

4. Discussion

In this systematic review, 30 studies related to the management of massive hemoptysis were included, of which 26 used bronchial artery embolization as a management method [45–54,56,57,59–64,66–72,74]. The 30 studies were observational retrospective cohort studies. As a result, no definitive conclusions can be made about the success of the methods for treating massive hemoptysis. The technical success of BAE ranges from 73.7% to 100%, while the clinical success ranges from 82.1% to 100%. This large variation depends on various factors, such as the technique and agents used, as well as the cause of the hemoptysis. Regarding the techniques, these initially include access to the vascular tree of the pulmonary parenchyma. This usually occurs via the femoral artery, although the transaxillary route has also been used. Embolization of the visible abnormal arteries then follows. The choice of the appropriate embolization factors is also important, as it has been found that they affect the success of the operation [35–37,75,76]. The most common agent is polyvinyl alcohol; however, a combination of agents has been found to slightly increase the technical success but significantly increase the clinical success [35–37,75,76]. Cheng et al. [45] showed that with the combination of embospheres and gelfoam particles, the technical success increased by 4.18%, while the clinical success jumped from 85.96% (without gelfoam particles) to 97.14%. It is worth mentioning the value of superselective arterial catheterization, which achieves the best results with the fewest possible complications [35–37,75,76].

The results of the meta-analysis demonstrate the success of BAE in the treatment of massive hemoptysis. Specifically, BAE scored a pooled technical success equal to 97.22% as well as a pooled clinical success equal to 92.46%. Therefore, BAE can with great ability both achieve arterial embolization and interrupt massive hemoptysis. However, the level of recurrence seems to be high (21.46%). Therefore, despite the immediate success of the intervention, the long-term success is limited due to the high recurrence numbers. Finally, mortality is limited to 3.5%, which also confirms the success of the intervention.

Surgical treatment is an alternative to BAE, which, however, is not minimally invasive, instead requiring a long operation with lobectomy of the bleeding lung segment. It is chosen in patients in whom temporary hemostasis or BAE will not produce a long-term effect, leading to rebleeding in a short period of time. It is a prerequisite that the patient is cardiorespiratorily fit for such an operation and that the bleeding is unilateral. Etiological therapy is chosen for respiratory diseases that do not cause anatomical damage and must be accompanied by respiratory support by administering oxygen [10,11,18]. It is the method of choice for conditions such as aspergilloma as well as for iatrogenic injuries that cause massive hemoptysis [77,78].

In the current systematic review, we defined massive hemoptysis as the expulsion of blood through the oral route in an amount exceeding 200 mL per twenty-four hours. In smaller amounts, hemoptysis is categorized as mild or moderate. In these cases, the patient is usually hemodynamically stable and the way to deal with hemoptysis changes, including treatment of the etiology that causes hemoptysis, and thus, together with the treatment of the cause of the hemoptysis, the hemoptysis itself is removed. However, it has been found that hemoptysis can be treated in these cases with the use of nebulized tranexamic acids. These are synthetic analogues of lysine with anti-fibrinolytic action. Specifically, they cause the suspension activation of plasminogen to plasmin and block the action of plasmin on fibrin. In the double-blind, randomized study by Wand et al., they were found to score 96% in the treatment of hemoptysis versus placebo, which achieved only 50%. This confirms the success of TAs in the management of mild-to-moderate hemoptysis. Also, the study showed that co-administration of antibiotics with TA does not increase the success of the intervention [14,79–82]

However, it has been found that moderate hemoptysis can potentially have the same prognosis of rebleeding as massive hemoptysis as well as the same mortality. For this reason, it is suggested that it be treated in the same way as the massive one. In other words, it is recommended to use BAE to treat it rather than etiological treatment or TA. In terms of success rates, these show the significant ability of BAE to manage moderate hemoptysis, scoring more than 96% and 94% for technical and clinical success, respectively [14,79–81].

Many factors have been implicated as risk factors for hemoptysis in the population. Initially, it was found that bronchiectasis is associated with an increased risk of hemoptysis, as well as hypertrophic bronchial arteries that are associated with heavier and faster hemodynamic instability [6,9,16,17,83,84]. As for hypertrophic arteries, it has been found that these are located in patients carrying the mutated BMPR2 gene. However, this mutation is not associated with an increased risk of hemoptysis but only with an increased frequency of bronchial artery hypertrophy. Smoking also increases the risk of developing hemoptysis, while anticoagulants and antiplatelet drugs increase both the risk of hemoptysis and the severity of this hemoptysis. Diabetes was also implicated as a risk factor, perhaps due to the vascular damage it causes. Hemoptysis occurs more often in males, while it occurs less often in diseases with a course between 1 and 5 years. Finally, with regard to massive hemoptysis, this occurs more often in diseases that affect two lobes or more, while the lower left lobe is less often involved in episodes of massive hemoptysis [6,8,9,11,83–86].

It has been found that, over time, the rate of clinical success decreases significantly. From the very first month after BAE, the clinical success rate can be significantly reduced due to the resulting rebleeding cases, which can be fatal. For this reason, long-term follow-up is considered useful in order to monitor the course of the patient's disease. In particular, certain conditions are associated with an increased risk of rebleeding in more than half of patients. Such diseases are bronchiectasis, aspergilloma, and especially lung tumors (primary and metastatic). In these cases, surgical treatment of hemoptysis should be discussed to reduce the risk of rebleeding. Many times, during follow-up, the need for re-interventions can be seen [45–54,56,57,59–64,66–72,74].

Rebleeding after BAE is the most frequent complication of surgery and determines the prognosis, as it can be fatal. Rebleeding occurs most frequently after the first month to the first year, with a mean day of occurrence of 293 postoperative days. It next most frequently appears in the first month after BAE. Rarely, however, rebleeding can occur after one year of BAE. However, these numbers vary quite a bit and are determined by the existence or not of risk factors. Such factors are diabetes, aspergilloma, and the existence of an arteriovenous shunt. In particular, with regard to aspergilloma, rebleeding can reach 100%, emphasizing the need for regular follow-up and discussion of surgical lobectomy if the patient is deemed cardiorespiratorily fit for such an operation [45–54,56,57,59–64,66–72,74].

Paresis, a serious complication, was reported twice in the included studies in this systematic review. Mishra et al. [71] documented monoparesis of the right lower extremity after BAE. This paresis was blamed on a small focal hyperintensity of the spinal cord due to a possible embolism of the spinal artery, as confirmed by magnetic resonance imaging. This complication requires physiotherapy that leads to partial-to-complete restoration of the damage. Other serious complications reported include aortic dissection, which occurred in one incident due to a fragile aortic wall. Two cases of cerebral infarction were also reported, one of which was attributed to infarction arising from the vertebral artery. This emphasizes the need for special care when embolizing near the vertebral artery.

Further investigation needs to be undertaken to find ways to treat massive hemoptysis non-invasively. Also, further investigation is required into how to prevent the complications of BAE, such as rebleeding, which occurs at a very high rate in some cases.

This research has certain limitations. One of them concerns the type of studies that were selected, these being retrospective observational cohort studies and not randomized controlled trials. This is due to the non-existence of other types of studies. Another constraint is the restriction of studies for inclusion to those written in the English language, which created publication bias, as well as the literature search being limited to a narrow period of time. Our systematic review does, however, have several strengths. Firstly, there is the rigorous methodology used according to the PRISMA guidelines and the exploration and reporting of all possible treatments of massive hemoptysis, in addition to only recent studies, i.e., those published in the last six years, having been selected.

5. Conclusions

In conclusion, massive hemoptysis is a life-threatening condition and is a frequent symptom of various respiratory diseases, such as COVID-19. Its treatment can be achieved in terms of technical and clinical success with the use of bronchial artery embolization. However, when this method is not indicated, the treatment of massive bleeding is achieved by using other equally effective methods. Complications appear in a large number of patients, the most common of which is chest discomfort. Rebleeding is a major problem, with massive bleeding occurring frequently, which can be fatal. Finally, mortality from massive hemoptysis occurs in a low percentage of patients, which reinforces the effectiveness of the methods of dealing with massive hemoptysis.

Author Contributions: Conceptualization, E.K. (Eleni Karlafti), L.K., G.T., G.K., C.S., A.M. and D.P.; methodology, E.K. (Evangelia Kotzakioulafi); software, D.T.; validation, E.K. (Eleni Karlafti), D.T., E.K. (Evangelia Kotzakioulafi) and S.N.; formal analysis, E.K. (Evangelia Kotzakioulafi) and D.T.; investigation, E.K. (Eleni Karlafti), D.T. and S.N.; resources, D.P., A.M. and C.S.; data curation, D.T. and S.N.; writing—original draft preparation, D.T., E.K. (Eleni Karlafti) and E.K. (Evangelia Kotzakioulafi); writing—review and editing, E.K. (Eleni Karlafti), D.T., E.K. (Evangelia Kotzakioulafi), L.K., G.T., G.K., C.S., A.M. and D.P.; visualization, E.K. (Evangelia Kotzakioulafi) and D.T.; supervision, C.S., G.K., A.M. and D.P.; project administration, C.S., G.K., A.M. and D.P. All authors have read and agreed to the published version of the manuscript.

Funding: This research received no external funding.

Institutional Review Board Statement: Not applicable.

Informed Consent Statement: Not applicable.

Data Availability Statement: No new data are created.

Conflicts of Interest: The authors declare no conflict of interest.

References

1. Pan, C.X.; Palathra, B.C.; Leo-To, W.F. Management of Respiratory Symptoms in Those with Serious Illness. *Med. Clin. N. Am.* **2020**, *104*, 455–470. [CrossRef] [PubMed]
2. Umakanthan, S.; Sahu, P.; Ranade, A.V.; Bukelo, M.M.; Rao, J.S.; Lf, A.-M.; Dahal, S.; Kumar, H.; Kv, D. Origin, transmission, diagnosis and management of coronavirus disease 2019 (COVID-19). *Postgrad Med. J.* **2020**, *96*, 753–758. [CrossRef] [PubMed]
3. Pradhan, M.; Shah, K.; Alexander, A.; Ajazuddin; Minz, S.; Singh, M.R.; Singh, D.; Yadav, K.; Chauhan, N.S. COVID-19: Clinical presentation and detection methods. *J. Immunoass. Immunochem.* **2022**, *43*, 1951291. [CrossRef] [PubMed]
4. Huang, C.; Wang, Y.; Li, X.; Ren, L.; Zhao, J.; Hu, Y.; Zhang, L.; Fan, G.; Xu, J.; Gu, X.; et al. Clinical features of patients infected with 2019 novel coronavirus in Wuhan, China. *Lancet* **2020**, *395*, 497–506. [CrossRef]
5. Dudha, M.; Lehrman, S.; Aronow, W.S.; Rosa, J. Hemoptysis: Diagnosis and treatment. *Compr. Ther.* **2009**, *35*, 139–149
6. Liippo, K.; Vasankari, T. Hemoptysis. *Duodecim* **2011**, *127*, 178–184.
7. Xi, Y.; Liu, D.; Yang, C.; Wu, X.; Nong, L.; He, W.; Liu, X.; Li, Y. Cause of massive hemoptysis in critical patients and the effect of bronchial artery embolization. *Zhonghua Wei Zhong Bing Ji Jiu Yi Xue* **2018**, *30*, 671–676. [CrossRef]
8. Noseworthy, T.W.; Anderson, B.J. Massive hemoptysis. *CMAJ* **1986**, *135*, 1097–1099.
9. Prey, B.; Francis, A.; Williams, J.; Krishnadasan, B. Evaluation and Treatment of Massive Hemoptysis. *Surg. Clin. N. Am.* **2022**, *102*, 465–481. [CrossRef]
10. Ittrich, H.; Bockhorn, M.; Klose, H.; Simon, M. The Diagnosis and Treatment of Hemoptysis. *Dtsch. Arztebl. Int.* **2017**, *114*, 371–381. [CrossRef]
11. Earwood, J.S.; Thompson, T.D. Hemoptysis: Evaluation and management. *Am. Fam. Physician.* **2015**, *91*, 243–249. [PubMed]
12. Aidé, M.A. Hemoptysis. *J. Bras Pneumol.* **2010**, *36*, 278–280. [CrossRef] [PubMed]
13. DiLeo, M.D.; Amedee, R.G.; Butcher, R.B. Hemoptysis and pseudohemoptysis: The patient expectorating blood. *Ear Nose Throat J.* **1995**, *74*, 822–824+826+828. [CrossRef] [PubMed]
14. Gavelli, F.; Patrucco, F.; Statti, G.; Balbo, P.E. Mild-to-moderate hemoptysis: A diagnostic and clinical challenge. *Minerva Med.* **2018**, *109*, 239–247. [CrossRef] [PubMed]
15. Larici, A.R.; Franchi, P.; Occhipinti, M.; Contegiacomo, A.; del Ciello, A.; Calandriello, L.; Storto, M.L.; Marano, R.; Bonomo, L. Diagnosis and management of hemoptysis. *Diagn. Interv. Radiol.* **2014**, *20*, 299–309. [CrossRef] [PubMed]
16. Bidwell, J.L.; Pachner, R.W. Hemoptysis: Diagnosis and management. *Am. Fam. Physician* **2005**, *72*, 1253–1260. [PubMed]
17. Khalil, A.; Fedida, B.; Parrot, A.; Haddad, S.; Fartoukh, M.; Carette, M.-F. Severe hemoptysis: From diagnosis to embolization. *Diagn. Interv. Imaging* **2015**, *96*, 775–788. [CrossRef]

18. Jin, F.; Li, Q.; Bai, C.; Wang, H.; Li, S.; Song, Y.; Zeng, Y.; Zhou, R.; Li, W.; Hu, C.; et al. Chinese Expert Recommendation for Diagnosis and Treatment of Massive Hemoptysis. *Respiration* **2020**, *99*, 83–92. [CrossRef]
19. Hsiao, E.I.; Kirsch, C.M.; Kagawa, F.T.; Wehner, J.H.; Jensen, W.A.; Baxter, R.B. Utility of fiberoptic bronchoscopy before bronchial artery embolization for massive hemoptysis. *Am. J. Roentgenol.* **2001**, *177*, 861–867. [CrossRef]
20. Sakr, L.; Dutau, H. Massive hemoptysis: An update on the role of bronchoscopy in diagnosis and management. *Respiration* **2010**, *80*, 38–58. [CrossRef]
21. Cahill, B.C.; Ingbar, D.H. Massive hemoptysis. Assessment and management. *Clin. Chest Med.* **1994**, *15*, 147–167. [CrossRef]
22. Cordovilla, R.; de Miguel, E.B.; Ares, A.N.; Povedano, F.J.C.; Ortega, I.H.; Merchán, R.J. Diagnóstico y tratamiento de la hemoptisis. *Arch Bronconeumol.* **2016**, *52*, 368–377. [CrossRef]
23. Wolfe, J.D.; Simmons, D.H. Hemoptysis: Diagnosis and management. *West J. Med.* **1977**, *127*, 383–390.
24. Revel, M.P.; Fournier, L.S.; Hennebicque, A.S.; Cuenod, C.A.; Meyer, G.; Reynaud, P.; Frija, G. Can CT replace bronchoscopy in the detection of the site and cause of bleeding in patients with large or massive hemoptysis? *Am. J. Roentgenol.* **2002**, *179*, 1217–1224. [CrossRef]
25. Yoon, W.; Kim, Y.H.; Kim, J.K.; Kim, Y.C.; Park, J.G.; Kang, H.K. Massive Hemoptysis: Prediction of Nonbronchial Systemic Arterial Supply with Chest CT. *Radiology* **2003**, *227*, 232–238. [CrossRef]
26. Solomonov, A.; Fruchter, O.; Zuckerman, T.; Brenner, B.; Yigla, M. Pulmonary hemorrhage: A novel mode of therapy. *Respir. Med.* **2009**, *103*, 1196–1200. [CrossRef]
27. Colchen, A.; Fischler, M. Emergency interventional bronchoscopies. *Rev. Pneumol. Clin.* **2011**, *67*, 209–213. [CrossRef]
28. Jean-Baptiste, E. Clinical assessment and management of massive hemoptysis. *Crit. Care Med.* **2000**, *28*, 1642–1647. [CrossRef]
29. Corey, R.; Hla, K.M. Major and massive hemoptysis: Reassessment of conservative management. *Am. J. Med. Sci.* **1987**, *294*, 301–309. [CrossRef]
30. Crocco, J.A.; Rooney, J.J.; Fankushen, D.S.; DiBenedetto, R.J.; Lyons, H.A. Massive hemoptysis. *Arch. Intern. Med.* **1968**, *121*, 495–498. [CrossRef] [PubMed]
31. Wahidi, M.M.; Rocha, A.T.; Hollingsworth, J.W.; Govert, J.A.; Feller-Kopman, D.; Ernst, A. Contraindications and safety of transbronchial lung biopsy via flexible bronchoscopy. A survey of pulmonologists and review of the literature. *Respiration* **2005**, *72*, 285–295. [CrossRef]
32. Papin, T.A.; Lynch, J.P.; Weg, J.G. Transbronchial biopsy in the thrombocytopenic patient. *Chest* **1985**, *88*, 549–552. [CrossRef]
33. Ernst, A.; Eberhardt, R.; Wahidi, M.; Becker, H.D.; Herth, F.J.F. Effect of routine clopidogrel use on bleeding complications after transbronchial biopsy in humans. *Chest* **2006**, *129*, 734–737. [CrossRef]
34. Dransfield, M.T.; Garver, R.I.; Weill, D. Standardized guidelines for surveillance bronchoscopy reduce complications in lung transplant recipients. *J. Heart Lung Transpl.* **2004**, *23*, 110–114. [CrossRef]
35. Lorenz, J.; Sheth, D.; Patel, J. Bronchial artery embolization. *Semin. Interv. Radiol.* **2012**, *29*, 155–160. [CrossRef]
36. Panda, A.; Bhalla, A.S.; Goyal, A. Bronchial artery embolization in hemoptysis: A systematic review. *Diagn. Interv. Radiol.* **2017**, *23*, 307–317. [CrossRef]
37. Kaufman, C.S.; Kwan, S.W. Bronchial Artery Embolization. *Semin. Interv. Radiol.* **2022**, *39*, 210–217. [CrossRef]
38. Page, M.J.; Moher, D.; Bossuyt, P.M.; Boutron, I.; Hoffmann, T.C.; Mulrow, C.D.; Shamseer, L.; Tetzlaff, J.M.; Akl, E.A.; Brennan, S.E.; et al. PRISMA 2020 explanation and elaboration: Updated guidance and exemplars for reporting systematic reviews. *BMJ* **2021**, *372*, n160. [CrossRef]
39. Ouzzani, M.; Hammady, H.; Fedorowicz, Z.; Elmagarmid, A. Rayyan—A web and mobile app for systematic reviews. *Syst. Rev.* **2016**, *5*, 210. [CrossRef] [PubMed]
40. Viechtbauer, W. Conducting Meta-Analyses in *R* with the metafor Package. *J. Stat. Softw.* **2010**, *36*, 1–48. [CrossRef]
41. Balduzzi, S.; Rücker, G.; Schwarzer, G. How to perform a meta-analysis with R: A practical tutorial. *Evid. Based Ment. Health* **2019**, *22*, 153–160. [CrossRef]
42. Egger, M.; Smith, G.D.; Schneider, M.; Minder, C. Bias in meta-analysis detected by a simple, graphical test. *BMJ* **1997**, *315*, 629–634. [CrossRef] [PubMed]
43. Higgins, J.P.T. Measuring inconsistency in meta-analyses. *BMJ* **2003**, *327*, 557–560. [CrossRef]
44. Higgins, J.; Green, S. *Cochrane Handbook for Systematic Reviews of Interventions Version 6.3 (Updated February 2022)*; The Cochrane Collaboration: London, UK, 2022.
45. Cheng, L.; Zhao, X.; Hu, X.; Huang, J.; Zhang, X. Safety and Efficacy Comparison of Embospheres and Gelfoam Particles in Bronchial Artery Embolization for Massive Hemoptysis. *Altern. Ther. Health Med.* **2023**, *29*, 298–301.
46. Li, H.; Ding, X.; Zhai, S.; Gao, K. A retrospective study on the management of massive hemoptysis by bronchial artery embolization: Risk factors associated with recurrence of hemoptysis. *BMC Pulm. Med.* **2023**, *23*, 87. [CrossRef] [PubMed]
47. An, J.; Dong, Y.; Niu, H. Application of the 5F JL4 Catheter in Bronchial Artery Embolization with the Opening in the Inferior Wall of the Aortic Arch. *Vasc. Endovasc. Surg.* **2023**, *57*, 379–385. [CrossRef]
48. Ando, T.; Kawashima, M.; Masuda, K.; Takeda, K.; Okuda, K.; Suzuki, J.; Ohshima, N.; Horibe, M.; Tamura, A.; Nagai, H.; et al. Exacerbation of chronic pulmonary aspergillosis was associated with a high rebleeding rate after bronchial artery embolization. *Respir. Investig.* **2019**, *57*, 260–267. [CrossRef] [PubMed]

49. Ishikawa, H.; Hara, M.; Ryuge, M.; Takafuji, J.; Youmoto, M.; Akira, M.; Nagasaka, Y.; Kabata, D.; Yamamoto, K.; Shintani, A. Efficacy and safety of super selective bronchial artery coil embolisation for haemoptysis: A single-centre retrospective observational study. *BMJ Open* **2017**, *7*, e014805. [CrossRef]
50. Le-Jun, F.; Sun, Y.; Fan, Y.; Jin, S. The effect of transcatheter bronchial artery embolization in five patients with bronchial artery aneurysm. *Postep. Kardiol Interwencyjnej* **2020**, *16*, 330–335. [CrossRef]
51. Springer, D.M.; Cofta, S.; Juszkat, R.; Żabicki, B.; Goździk-Spychalska, J.; Nowicka, A.; Winiarska, H.; Batura-Gabryel, H. The effectiveness of bronchial artery embolisation in patients with haemoptysis. *Adv. Respir. Med.* **2018**, *86*, 220–226. [CrossRef]
52. Flight, W.G.; Barry, P.J.; Bright-Thomas, R.J.; Butterfield, S.; Ashleigh, R.; Jones, A.M. Outcomes Following Bronchial Artery Embolisation for Haemoptysis in Cystic Fibrosis. *Cardiovasc. Interv. Radiol.* **2017**, *40*, 1164–1168. [CrossRef] [PubMed]
53. Frood, R.; Karthik, S.; Mirsadraee, S.; Clifton, I.; Flood, K.; McPherson, S.J. Bronchial Artery Embolisation for Massive Haemoptysis: Immediate and Long-Term Outcomes-A Retrospective Study. *Pulm. Ther.* **2020**, *6*, 107–117. [CrossRef] [PubMed]
54. Lee, Y.; Lee, M.; Hur, S.; Kim, H.-C.; Jae, H.J.; Chung, J.W.; Choi, J.W. Bronchial and non-bronchial systemic artery embolization with transradial access in patients with hemoptysis. *Diagn. Interv. Radiol.* **2022**, *28*, 359–363. [CrossRef] [PubMed]
55. Lal, A.; Bansal, A.; Chaluvashetty, S.B.; Sandhu, M.S.; Gorsi, U. Percutaneous transthoracic embolisation for massive haemoptysis secondary to peripheral pulmonary artery pseudoaneurysms. *Eur. Radiol.* **2021**, *31*, 2183–2190. [CrossRef] [PubMed]
56. Kucukay, F.; Topcuoglu, O.M.; Alpar, A.; Altay, Ç.M.; Kucukay, M.B.; Ozbulbul, N.I. Bronchial Artery Embolization with Large Sized (700–900 μm) Tris-acryl Microspheres (Embosphere) for Massive Hemoptysis: Long-Term Results (Clinical Research). *Cardiovasc. Interv. Radiol.* **2018**, *41*, 225–230. [CrossRef] [PubMed]
57. Floridi, C.; Boscarato, P.; Ventura, C.; Bruno, A.; Rossini, N.; Baldassari, M.; Lanza, C.; Fabrizzi, B.; Candelari, R.; Giovagnoni, A. Role of Bronchial Artery Embolization as Early Treatment Option in Stable Cystic Fibrosis Patients with Sub-Massive Hemoptysis: Personal Experience and Literature Review. *J. Clin. Med.* **2022**, *11*, 6432. [CrossRef]
58. Al-Samkari, H.; Shin, K.; Cardoni, L.; Pighetti, E.H.; Rits, S.; McMahon, L.; Perkins, R.; Uluer, A.; Connors, J.M. Antifibrinolytic Agents for Hemoptysis Management in Adults with Cystic Fibrosis. *Chest* **2019**, *155*, 1226–1233. [CrossRef]
59. Seki, A.; Shimono, C. Transarterial chemoembolization for management of hemoptysis: Initial experience in advanced primary lung cancer patients. *Jpn. J. Radiol.* **2017**, *35*, 495–504. [CrossRef]
60. Han, K.; Yoon, K.W.; Kim, J.H.; Kim, G.M. Bronchial Artery Embolization for Hemoptysis in Primary Lung Cancer: A Retrospective Review of 84 Patients. *J. Vasc. Interv. Radiol.* **2019**, *30*, 428–434. [CrossRef]
61. Xiaobing, L.; Meipan, Y.; Pengfei, X.; Yue, Z.; Ying, L.; Xiangnan, L.; Yu, Q.; Yaozhen, M.; Chunxia, L.; Gang, W. Bronchial Artery Chemoembolization for Hemoptysis in Advanced Primary Lung Cancer. *Clin. Lung Cancer* **2022**, *23*, e203–e209. [CrossRef]
62. Miyano, Y.; Kanzaki, M.; Onuki, T. Bronchial artery embolization: First-line option for managing massive hemoptysis. *Asian Cardiovasc. Thorac. Ann.* **2017**, *25*, 618–622. [CrossRef] [PubMed]
63. Marcelin, C.; Soussan, J.; Desmots, F.; Gaubert, J.-Y.; Vidal, V.; Bartoli, J.M.; Izaaryene, J. Outcomes of Pulmonary Artery Embolization and Stent Graft Placement for the Treatment of Hemoptysis Caused by Lung Tumors. *J. Vasc. Interv. Radiol.* **2018**, *29*, 975–980. [CrossRef]
64. Keshmiri, M.S.; Shafaghi, S.; Sharif-Kashani, B.; Sadoughi, A.; Ghorbani, F.; Naghashzadeh, F.; Abedini, A. Preemptive non-selective bronchial artery angioembolization to reduce recurrence rate of hemoptysis. *Multidiscip Respir. Med.* **2020**, *15*, 723. [CrossRef]
65. Mehta, R.M.; Godara, R.; Bhat, R.S.; Loknath, C.; Singla, A. A Novel Technique for the Management of Massive Hemoptysis: The Customized Endobronchial Silicone Blocker. *Innovations* **2020**, *15*, 142–147. [CrossRef]
66. MKolu; Kurtuluş, Ş.; Dere, O.; Yurttutan, N.; Yıldırım, I.O. Embolization with more diluted glue-lipiodol in patients with massive hemoptysis: Single center experience results. *Eur. Rev. Med. Pharmacol. Sci.* **2022**, *26*, 1543–1548. [CrossRef]
67. Ando, T.; Kawashima, M.; Masuda, K.; Takeda, K.; Okuda, K.; Suzuki, J.; Ohshima, N.; Matsui, H.; Tamura, A.; Nagai, H.; et al. Clinical and Angiographic Characteristics of 35 Patients with Cryptogenic Hemoptysis. *Chest* **2017**, *152*, 1008–1014. [CrossRef] [PubMed]
68. Fu, Z.; Liang, Y.; Zhao, W.; Tian, J.; Cai, F.; Zhang, X. Safety and efficacy of transcatheter embolization in patients with massive hemoptysis due to intercostal pulmonary venous shunts. *Radiol. Med.* **2019**, *124*, 588–594. [CrossRef] [PubMed]
69. Seyyedi, S.R.; Sadeghipour, P.; Sadr, M.; Shafe, O.; Moosavi, J.; Aloosh, O.; Abedini, A.; Sharif-Kashani, B. Outcomes and Complications of Bronchial Angioembolization in Patients with Massive Hemoptysis. *Tanaffos* **2019**, *18*, 310–314.
70. Da Silveira, M.A.P.; da Silveira, P.A.P.; Beltrami, F.G.; Scaffaro, L.A.; Dalcin, P.d.T.R. Clinical outcomes of cystic fibrosis patients with hemoptysis treated with bronchial artery embolization. *J. Bras. Pneumol.* **2021**, *47*, e20200557. [CrossRef]
71. Mishra, A.; Mathur, A.; Pathak, K.; Katoch, C.D.S.; Khera, A. Bronchial artery embolization in treatment of hemoptysis: Treatment efficacy and complications at a tertiary care chest centre. *Med. J. Armed Forces India* **2018**, *74*, 352–357. [CrossRef]
72. Clements, W.; Venn, G.; McGiffin, D.; Moriarty, H.K.; Joseph, T.; Goh, G.S.; Whitford, H.; Keating, D. Chronic Thromboembolic Pulmonary Hypertension (CTEPH) and massive hemoptysis: The rationale for bronchial artery embolization. *Respir. Med.* **2022**, *195*, 106784. [CrossRef] [PubMed]
73. Yang, Q.; Luo, L.C.; Wei, H.; Yi, Q.; Luo, W. Dual-vessel intervention treatment for massive hemoptysis caused by lung cavitary lesions. *Eur. J. Radiol.* **2022**, *154*, 110448. [CrossRef]
74. Abid, N.; Loukil, M.; Mokni, A.; Badri, I.; Bouzaidi, K.; Ghrairi, H. Outcomes of bronchial artery embolization for the management of hemoptysis. *Tunis Med.* **2021**, *99*, 264–268. [PubMed]

75. Temel, U.; Akgul, A.G.; Dogan, S. Bronchial Artery Embolization, an Increasingly Used Method for Hemoptysis; Treatment and Avoidance. *Sisli. Etfal. Hastan. Tıp. Bul.* **2020**, *54*, 313–319. [CrossRef] [PubMed]
76. Burke, C.T.; Mauro, M.A. Bronchial artery embolization. *Semin. Interv. Radiol.* **2004**, *21*, 43–48. [CrossRef] [PubMed]
77. Kiral, H.; Evman, S.; Tezel, C.; Alpay, L.; Lacin, T.; Baysungur, V.; Yalcinkaya, I. Pulmonary resection in the treatment of life-threatening hemoptysis. *Ann. Thorac Cardiovasc. Surg.* **2015**, *21*, 125–131. [CrossRef] [PubMed]
78. Nakajima, T.; Yoshino, I. Massive Hemoptysis; Clinical Approach and Surgical Treatment. *Kyobu Geka* **2015**, *68*, 665–670.
79. Ketai, L.H.; Mohammed, T.-L.H.; Kirsch, J.; Kanne, J.P.; Chung, J.H.; Donnelly, E.F.; Ginsburg, M.E.; Heitkamp, D.E.; Henry, T.S.; Kazerooni, E.A.; et al. ACR appropriateness criteria® hemoptysis. *J. Thorac Imaging* **2014**, *29*, W19–W22. [CrossRef]
80. Johnson, J.L. Manifestations of hemoptysis. How to manage minor, moderate, and massive bleeding. *Postgrad Med.* **2002**, *112*, 101–106+108–109+113. [CrossRef]
81. Lee, M.K.; Kim, S.; Yong, S.J.; Shin, K.C.; Kim, H.S.; Yu, T.; Choi, E.H.; Lee, W. Moderate hemoptysis: Recurrent hemoptysis and mortality according to bronchial artery embolization. *Clin. Respir. J.* **2015**, *9*, 53–64. [CrossRef]
82. Wand, O.; Guber, E.; Guber, A.; Shochet, G.E.; Israeli-Shani, L.; Shitrit, D. Inhaled Tranexamic Acid for Hemoptysis Treatment. *Chest* **2018**, *154*, 1379–1384. [CrossRef] [PubMed]
83. Luo, L.; Luo, J.; Jiang, Y. A retrospective analysis of risk factors for massive hemoptysis in patients with bronchiectasis. *BMC Pulm. Med.* **2022**, *22*, 214. [CrossRef] [PubMed]
84. Tio, D.; Leter, E.; Boerrigter, B.; Boonstra, A.; Vonk-Noordegraaf, A.; Bogaard, H.J. Risk factors for hemoptysis in idiopathic and hereditary pulmonary arterial hypertension. *PLoS ONE* **2013**, *8*, e78132. [CrossRef] [PubMed]
85. Rali, P.; Gandhi, V.; Tariq, C. Massive Hemoptysis. *Crit. Care Nurs. Q* **2016**, *39*, 139–147. [CrossRef]
86. Kim, T.H.; Koo, H.J.; Lim, C.-M.; Hong, S.-B.; Huh, J.W.; Jo, K.W.; Shim, T.S.; Kim, W.S.; Koh, Y. Risk factors of severe hemoptysis in patients with fungus ball. *J. Thorac Dis.* **2019**, *11*, 4249–4257. [CrossRef]

MDPI AG
Grosspeteranlage 5
4052 Basel
Switzerland
Tel.: +41 61 683 77 34

Journal of Personalized Medicine Editorial Office
E-mail: jpm@mdpi.com
www.mdpi.com/journal/jpm